# Understanding BACK AND NECK PAIN

## A Yogic Perspective

What doctors don't have time to explain

**Yogāchārya Vinay Siddaiah**

ISBN
Paperback 979-8-90362-380-8
Hardcase 979-8-90431-692-1

# CONTENTS

*Foreword*

# A HOLISTIC YOGIC PERSPECTIVE ON PAIN AND HEALING

Lifestyle-related disorders are increasing rapidly across the world, affecting both physical and mental well-being. Among these conditions, back and neck pain have emerged as major contributors to reduced productivity, and diminished quality of life. These problems affect individuals across professions and age groups, reflecting the profound changes in lifestyle, work patterns, and stress levels in modern society.

Advances in medical science have provided sophisticated tools for diagnosis and acute management. However, persistent musculoskeletal pain cannot always be explained solely by structural abnormalities. Increasing scientific evidence indicates that chronic pain is influenced by multiple factors, including posture, movement habits, neuromuscular coordination, stress, emotional state, and lifestyle patterns. Therefore, a purely structural approach often remains incomplete.

Yoga offers a holistic framework to understand and address this complexity. The yogic view considers the human being as an integrated personality. The classical Panchakosha model, described in the Upanishadic tradition, beautifully illustrates this understanding. It explains how human experience unfolds across multiple layers of existence, from the physical body to subtler dimensions of life. When imbalance arises in any of these layers, it may manifest as discomfort or disease in the body. Restoration of harmony across these dimensions forms the foundation of yogic healing.

Over the past several decades, research in Yoga therapy, including studies conducted at S-VYASA, has demonstrated the effectiveness of integrated Yoga practices in managing chronic pain conditions. Yogic techniques have been shown to improve autonomic balance, reduce muscular tension, enhance body awareness, and promote psychological resilience. These findings support the classical understanding that regulation of the mind and breath plays a central role in restoring physical well-being.

In this context, this book by Vinay Siddaiah is a valuable contribution. Drawing from his experience as a Yoga therapist and teacher, he presents a clear and systematic understanding of back and neck pain. The author explains how biomechanics, nervous system responses, lifestyle patterns, and emotional influences together shape the experience of pain. Through clear explanations and helpful illustrations, the book enables readers to understand these mechanisms in a practical and accessible manner.

Importantly, the book guides readers beyond fear and structural fixation toward an appreciation of the body's inherent intelligence and capacity for adaptation.

The strength of this work lies in its integrative perspective. It bridges traditional yogic wisdom with contemporary scientific insights and emphasizes awareness, balanced movement, breath regulation, and mindful living as essential components of healing. By presenting Yoga not merely as physical exercise but as a comprehensive approach to self-regulation and harmony, the author offers readers a practical pathway toward recovery and long-term well-being.

This book will be useful not only to individuals suffering from back and neck pain, but also to Yoga therapists, healthcare professionals, and all those interested in an integrated approach to health.

May this work inspire a deeper understanding of the body–mind connection and encourage readers to move from fear to understanding, thereby transforming their relationship with pain.

With blessings and best wishes,

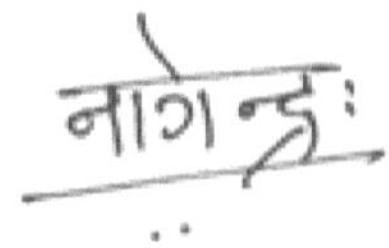

**Dr. H. R. Nagendra**
President, VYASA

*Foreword*

# THE LIVING TEMPLE OF THE HUMAN SPINE

Namaste,

It gives me immense joy to pen a few words for this thoughtful work by my dear student and colleague, Yoga Chikitsa Acharya Vinay Siddaiah. When a sincere sadhaka reflects deeply on the suffering of humanity and seeks answers through the timeless wisdom of Yoga, such a book naturally arises. This text on *Understanding Back and Neck Pain: A Yogic Perspective* is not merely a manual about the spine—it is a gentle reminder that the human being must be understood as an integrated whole.

Modern society has become extremely efficient at studying the body as if it were a machine composed of replaceable parts. In this mechanical model, the back becomes a structure of bones and discs, the neck a set of joints and muscles, and pain something to be suppressed through medication or corrected through procedures. Yet Yoga reminds us that the human being is far more than this mechanical arrangement. We are a living, conscious, psycho-physiological organism, where body, breath, mind and spirit interact continuously.

When this deeper understanding is forgotten, we fall prey to what may be called the illusion of treatment. We attempt to chase symptoms rather than understand the disharmony that gave rise to them. Yogic wisdom reminds us that true healing begins when we search for the root cause of the disorder rather than merely its outward manifestation. The ancient Tamil sage Tiruvalluvar beautifully advised us to *look for the disease, look for the primary cause and then treat it.*

Back and neck pain provide a perfect example of this misunderstanding. Many individuals live in fear after seeing an MRI report mentioning disc bulges, degeneration or alignment changes. Yet, the presence of a structural change does not automatically condemn one to a lifetime of suffering. The body is not a static structure; it is a dynamic system constantly adapting to the way we live, breathe, think and move. Yoga views health not as a fixed state but as a dynamic continuum where the individual can move toward balance and harmony.

In the yogic tradition, the spine is revered as the Brahma Danda—the staff of the Divine. It forms the central axis around which the entire human structure is organized. The limbs attach to this axial column, and within it runs the spinal cord carrying messages between the brain and every organ of the body. To maintain the integrity of this central axis is therefore essential not only for physical comfort but for the harmonious functioning of the entire being.

From a Yogic perspective, the practices of asana, pranayama and conscious living are designed to nurture this central column of life. Every classical posture—whether stretching upward, bending forward, extending backward or twisting gently—works to mobilize and revitalize the spine. Through these movements we restore elasticity to tissues, balance muscular activity and stimulate circulation in the vital neural pathways.

An interesting point often overlooked in conventional approaches is that the neck and the back are not separate entities. They are different expressions of the same spinal continuum. A disturbance in one segment inevitably influences the others. A stiff thoracic region may overload the cervical spine; a restricted hip may transmit strain upward through the lumbar area. Yoga therefore approaches the spine as a unified functional system, not as isolated compartments.

The regular practice of yogic movements provides something remarkably valuable—a gentle and intelligent self-traction of the spine. In hospitals, traction may be applied through elaborate equipment using weights and pulleys. Yet the body itself possesses the capacity to create this therapeutic elongation when the practitioner stretches mindfully in appropriate postures. At the same time, muscles receive an isometric conditioning that combines strength with deep relaxation. This dual action of effort and ease reflects the classical yogic principle of *sthira and sukha*—steadiness combined with comfort.

However, Yoga must never be reduced to a mechanical set of exercises. True Yoga therapy recognizes that pain is not merely a structural event but also a neurophysiological and psychological experience. Our nervous system constantly interprets signals from the body and the environment, deciding whether we are safe or threatened. When the system perceives threat, protective tension arises in muscles and connective tissues, amplifying the sensation of pain.

For this reason, the breath becomes the first gateway to healing. Conscious breathing calms the autonomic nervous system, bringing balance between sympathetic arousal and parasympathetic restoration. As the breath deepens and lengthens, the body begins to feel safe again. Only in this state of safety can genuine structural correction or rehabilitation take place.

This book also brings attention to the fascinating concepts of fascial connectivity and tensegrity, ideas that resonate beautifully with yogic insights that the body functions as an interconnected web rather than isolated parts. A distortion in the foot, prolonged sitting, or habitual use of digital devices may create subtle tensions that ripple upward through the entire structure, eventually manifesting as neck or back pain. Such understanding echoes the yogic concept of *yuj*—the fundamental principle of union and interconnectedness.

Equally important is the recognition that the body possesses a remarkable capacity for adaptation and transformation. What appears fixed today may change tomorrow through appropriate stimulus and awareness. Yoga therefore encourages us to replace fear with curiosity, rigidity with adaptability, and passivity with conscious participation in our own healing process.

Healing, however, is rarely a straight line. It is more like a journey from imbalance toward harmony, from fear toward confidence, and from fragmentation toward integration. Yoga Chikitsa serves as a compassionate support in this journey, empowering individuals to rediscover the inherent intelligence of their own bodies.

My dear Vinay has attempted in this work to build a bridge—between ancient yogic wisdom and contemporary scientific understanding, between structural anatomy and functional awareness, and most importantly between knowledge and practice. Such integrative thinking is essential if Yoga is to retain its authenticity while remaining relevant in the modern world.

I encourage readers to approach this book not merely with analytical intellect but with inner awareness. Reflect on your posture, your breathing, your daily habits and your relationship with your own body. In doing so, you may discover that the spine is not merely a column of bones but truly a living temple of consciousness.

May this work inspire you to care for this sacred axis of life and to cultivate that beautiful state described in our yogic tradition as sukha sthanam—a dynamic sense of well-being in body, mind and spirit.

With blessings for health, harmony and conscious evolution.

Be Yoga.

---

Yoga Chikitsa Ratna, Puduvai Kalaimamani

Yogacharya Dr. Ananda Balayogi Bhavanani, DSc (Yoga), C-IAYT

- Ashram Acharya and Chairman ICYER Ananda Ashram, Pondicherry (www.icyer.com)
- Founder Guru Sannidhi Yoga (www.sannidhi.yoga) & GITA (www.rishiculture.com)
- Director and Professor, Institute of Salutogenesis and Complementary Medicine, Sri Balaji Vidyapeeth, Pondicherry. (www.sbvu.ac.in/iscm)

# ACKNOWLEDGEMENTS

No journey unfolds in isolation. The ideas in this book are the result of many years of learning, questioning, teaching, observing, and receiving guidance from many individuals who shaped my understanding along the way.

I offer my deepest gratitude to Padma Shri Dr. H. R. Nagendra, President of VYASA and former Chancellor of S-VYASA Yoga University, for kindly agreeing to write the foreword for this book. His lifelong contribution to integrating Yoga with modern scientific understanding has inspired countless students of Yoga across the world, including me. His encouragement and guidance mean a great deal to me.

I am equally grateful to my teacher Dr. Ananda Balayogi Bhavanani of Ananda Ashram for graciously writing the foreword for this book. His tireless work in promoting Yoga therapy and his ability to bridge traditional Yogic wisdom with modern medical understanding have been deeply inspiring.

My journey into Yoga began not through philosophy but through pain. I must acknowledge my mountaineering teacher, whose advice during a difficult climb changed the direction of my life. When he told me that if I wanted to continue climbing mountains I must first fix my back, I did not realize that this suggestion would lead me to a lifelong exploration of Yoga.

My first Yoga teacher, Shri Sanjay Gurvekar, played a pivotal role in this journey. Under his guidance I began my first Yoga practice during my time at Intel. It was his trust in asking me to take over his class in 2010 that led me to begin teaching Yoga.

I would also like to thank Shri Raghavendra Shenoy, Dr. S. N. Omkar, Shri Kartik Chaitanya, and Shri Rangaji, from whom I learned many aspects of Yoga during my early years of exploration. I also acknowledge Shri Sharat Arora, from whom I had the opportunity to learn during my time in Dharamshala. His teachings deepened my understanding of discipline and exploration.

My understanding of the human body deepened through the generosity of Dr. Gladson Johnson, one of the finest sports physiotherapists in Bangalore. Spending weekends at his clinic observing, learning anatomy and physiology, and understanding body mechanics opened an important dimension in my study of Yoga.

I am also grateful to my friend Dr. Swaroop R, who helped me explore the philosophical depth of Yoga. Many evenings spent discussing Yogic philosophy with him helped me appreciate that Yoga cannot be understood through anatomy alone.

I offer my sincere gratitude to S-VYASA Yoga University, where I completed my master's degree in Yoga therapy. The training and academic exposure I received there strengthened my understanding of Yoga as a therapeutic discipline.

My academic journey was further enriched during my MTech at IIT Hyderabad in Heritage Science and Technology, where I explored technology in relation to Yoga and traditional knowledge systems. I am grateful to my professors at both S-VYASA University and IIT Hyderabad for encouraging a scientific approach toward understanding Yoga and its broader cultural and technological context.

Corporate organizations I worked with, including Intel and Sandisk, supported my journey by giving me the freedom to explore Yoga teaching while continuing my work in technology. Their support played an important role in shaping my journey as a teacher.

The journey of Yogavijnana would not have been possible without the trust and enthusiasm of the entire Yogavijnana family. Every class, question, and experience shared by students contributed to the insights that shaped this book. Teaching has been my greatest teacher.

I am grateful to the institutions that provided opportunities for me to share my understanding of Yoga and Yoga therapy. I would like to particularly acknowledge The Yoga Institute, Mumbai, and Kathmandu University, Nepal, for inviting me to contribute as a teacher. I also extend my sincere thanks to the Indian Yoga Association and my friends there for their continued encouragement and support.

My sincere thanks to Dr. Veena R., Akshatha Rao, Prathibha Chandra, Vijaya Siddaiah, and Uttam Kumar for reviewing the manuscript and offering thoughtful feedback that helped refine this book. Thanks to Vinutha V S for the cover design.

I would also like to express my heartfelt gratitude to my father, Siddaiah K, whose quiet trust and encouragement during the early stages of my journey gave me the confidence to continue exploring this path. I am equally grateful to my mother, Padma, for her constant care, patience, and support throughout this journey.

My deepest gratitude goes to my family, who showed patience and understanding during the times I chose to step away from a conventional corporate career to pursue Yoga more fully. Their support made it possible for me to remain committed to this path.

I am also thankful to my friends whose encouragement supported me through different stages of this journey.

Above all, I remain deeply grateful to the tradition of Yoga itself. Even today, I consider myself first and foremost a student of Yoga. This book is simply an attempt to share what I have learned so far in this ongoing journey.

Vinay Siddaiah
Founder, Yogavijnana (www.yogavijnana.in)
Bangalore

**Illustration Credits**

The diagrams and conceptual illustrations in this book were created with the assistance of AI-based image generation tools and subsequently refined by the author to accurately represent the concepts discussed.

PART I

# RETHINKING PAIN: MOVING BEYOND THE OBVIOUS

# INTRODUCTION

Physical pain is one of the most common experiences of modern life. Back pain, neck pain, joint discomfort, and recurring muscular aches affect people across age groups, professions, and lifestyles. For many, pain becomes a constant companion, shaping daily choices and quietly limiting freedom of movement. Yet despite its prevalence, pain is often approached in fragmented and incomplete ways.

This book begins with back pain not because it is the only form of physical pain that matters, but because it reveals the body's adaptive intelligence with particular clarity. The back sits at the center of movement, and balance. When strain, compensation, or imbalance develops anywhere in the body, it often finds expression in the spine. For this reason, back pain becomes a natural entry point for understanding how physical pain emerges, adapts, and persists.

As the exploration unfolds, it becomes evident that the same principles governing back pain also apply to neck pain, shoulder discomfort, joint issues, and many other forms of chronic physical pain. The locations may differ, but the underlying processes remain the same. What the body learns in one region is often reflected elsewhere.

Modern approaches to pain frequently focus on structure. Discs, joints, bones, and alignment receive primary attention, often guided by imaging and diagnostic reports. While these tools are valuable, they capture only part of the story. Pain does not arise from structure alone. It emerges from the interaction of posture, movement patterns, muscle tone, nervous system regulation, emotional state, and the body's ongoing capacity to adapt.

This book offers a yogic perspective on physical pain, not as an alternative to medicine, but as a complementary way of understanding the human system. Yoga, in its classical sense, is not merely a collection of asana to be performed or prescribed. It is a method of observation. A way of understanding how body, breath, mind, and awareness function together as an integrated whole. Through this lens, pain is not treated as an isolated symptom to be eliminated, but as meaningful feedback from an intelligent system that has adapted under specific conditions.

It is important to be clear about what this book is *not*. This is not a manual of prescribed asana or fixed therapeutic sequences. Practices cannot be standardized because pain is never standardized in the body. A posture that supports one person may aggravate pain in another. Meaningful practice must be learned experimentally and experientially, guided with sensitivity, and adapted to individual needs under the observation of an experienced teacher.

The intention here is not to tell you *what to do*, but to help you understand *why* certain approaches help and others do not.

The chapters that follow explore biomechanics, anatomy, posture, nervous system responses, emotional influence, and habitual patterns using language accessible to those without medical training. Analogies are used to simplify complex ideas. Case studies drawn from real experience illustrate how similar structural findings can lead to very different outcomes. Throughout the book, the emphasis is placed on understanding rather than quick fixes.

The aim is not to promise instant relief or universal solutions. Instead, this book invites a shift in perspective. When we understand how the body learns, compensates, and adapts, pain becomes less mysterious. Choices become clearer, and interventions become more thoughtful. Healing reveals itself as a process rather than a single event.

Although doctors may not always have the time to explore these dimensions within the constraints of clinical practice, they remain essential for anyone seeking lasting change. This book is an attempt to articulate those missing conversations, bridging modern understanding with timeless yogic insight.

What follows is an exploration of physical pain as a multidimensional experience. The back and neck will guide us, but the lessons extend far beyond them. Ultimately, this is a book about learning to listen to the body, not as a machine that breaks down, but as a living system that continuously responds to how it is used, held, and understood.

# WHY I AM WRITING THIS BOOK?

Honestly, this book was not planned.

It did not begin as a project, a proposal, or an ambition to author a text. It emerged slowly, first through the firsthand experience of going through the back pain, and then professionally as a Yoga therapist listening to people in pain, watching patterns repeat themselves, and noticing how often the same misunderstandings surfaced across many people of different ages, and diagnoses.

Over the years, I have met people who came to me for therapy after being advised surgery, people who came after surgery, and people who came confused by medical reports that did not match their living experience. Many arrived carrying fear, some with frustration, and some with a quiet resignation that pain was now a permanent part of their lives. What struck me was not just the presence of pain, but the absence of understanding.

People were told *what* was wrong, but rarely helped to understand *why* it was happening or *how* their body had arrived there. Imaging reports, labels, and diagnoses often replaced conversation. Time constraints limited deeper exploration and as a result, many people carried a fragmented understanding of their own bodies.

This book is an attempt to fill that gap.

It is not written in opposition to medicine, nor does it claim that Yoga is an universal solution. Instead, it seeks to offer a broader lens. A way of seeing pain not as an isolated structural problem, but as a multidimensional experience shaped by movement, posture, nervous system patterns, emotions, habits, and time.

I am writing this book because I have seen that when people understand their bodies better, fear reduces. When fear reduces, movement becomes possible. When movement becomes conscious, healing often begins in ways that need not be forced but can be supported.

This book is an invitation to that understanding.

# MY ACCIDENTAL JOURNEY INTO YOGA AND BACK PAIN

I did not grow up practicing Yoga.

Until the end of my graduation, Yoga was not part of my life in any meaningful way. I was physically active, involved in sports, and later drawn toward mountaineering and climbing. At the same time, I was building a corporate career that demanded long hours of sitting and irregular physical routines. These two extremes, intense physical challenge on one side and prolonged inactivity on the other, eventually converged in the form of back pain.

The trigger that brought me to Yoga was not philosophical curiosity or spiritual seeking but rather it was a physical necessity.

A mountaineering teacher once told me very clearly, "If you want to continue climbing, go fix your back and come back. You can do some Yoga, it will help" That sentence became my motivation to attend my first Yoga class.

Within a few months of practice, I experienced tangible improvement. The pain reduced, movement felt freer, and strength returned. But instead of stopping there, a deeper question arose. With a background in engineering, who questioned and analyzed everything, I wanted to understand *how* this had worked. What exactly had changed? Why did certain practices help my back while other approaches did not?

This curiosity led me to study under multiple teachers, many rooted in the Iyengar tradition, and later started studying anatomy and physiology under the guidance of a sports physiotherapist. Over time, it became clear that anatomy alone did not explain everything. The philosophical foundations of Yoga, particularly its understanding of mind, breath, and awareness, were equally essential.

Teaching entered my life unexpectedly. When my first teacher had to relocate, he asked me to take over his classes temporarily. I resisted at first, convinced I was not qualified. His response was simple. "Try it for a month."

That month changed everything.

Teaching forced me to articulate what I had only felt intuitively. Questions from students exposed gaps in my understanding and pushed me to study more deeply. Eventually, my engagement with Yoga grew to a point where it became impossible to keep it separate for the rest of my life.

I took a break from my career, spent extended time in the Himalayas, deepened my personal practice, and eventually made the decision to step away from corporate life entirely. What began as a response to back pain slowly transformed into a lifelong commitment to learning, practicing, and teaching Yoga.

Yogavijnana- center for Yoga, Therapy and Research, was born not as an institution, but as a continuation of this journey. Over the years, teaching thousands of students, working in therapeutic settings, engaging with research, and participating in education and certification roles, one thought remained constant.

I am, first and foremost, a student.

Even today, I spend more time studying and reflecting than teaching. This book arises from that ongoing inquiry. It is not a conclusion, but a sharing of what has been learned so far, offered with humility and hope that it may help others relate to their bodies with greater clarity and confidence.

# WHY BACK OR NECK PAIN IS NOT SIMPLE?

Back or Neck pain is often spoken about as if it were a single problem with a clear cause and a clear solution. A disc bulge, a muscle strain, a poor posture, or a weak back are commonly offered explanations. Yet for anyone who has lived with back pain or worked closely with those who do, this simplicity quickly dissolves.

Two people can have similar pain but very different diagnoses. Two people can have similar MRI findings but completely different experiences of discomfort. One person may recover quickly, while another continues to suffer for years despite treatment. These contradictions reveal an important truth. Back or Neck pain is not a single condition. It is an experience shaped by many interacting factors.

One of the reasons back or neck pain feels so confusing is that it does not always follow a predictable pattern. Pain may appear all of a sudden without any clear injury. It may persist even after tissues have healed. It may shift location, disappear for a while, and return unexpectedly. Sometimes pain is intense despite minimal findings on imaging such as MRI. At other times, significant structural changes exist without any pain at all.

This inconsistency often leads to frustration. Patients search for answers. They go on taking different opinions and multiple imaging. Therapies are tried and abandoned. Each approach may offer partial relief, yet the underlying question remains unanswered. Why does the pain behave this way?

Part of the difficulty lies in how the body is often understood. The spine is frequently treated as a mechanical structure made up of bones and discs. While this is anatomically correct, it is incomplete. Pain is not produced by the structure alone. It arises from how the structure is used, loaded, protected, compensated for, and perceived by the nervous system. A small structural change may produce significant pain if the surrounding system is sensitive or strained. A larger structural change may produce no pain if the system is well supported and adaptable.

Modern medicine offers powerful tools for visualizing the body, especially through imaging techniques such as MRI. These tools have greatly improved our understanding of anatomy. However, they also carry a limitation. They show what the body looks like, not how it functions. They capture structure, not experience.

This gap between image and experience is where much confusion about back or neck pain begins. When pain is explained primarily through images, treatments may focus on correcting what is seen rather than understanding how the body is responding. This can lead to interventions that address structure while leaving underlying patterns unchanged.

From a yogic perspective, the body is not viewed as a collection of isolated parts but as an integrated whole. Movement, breath, posture, attention, mindset and emotional state are all part of one system. Pain is understood as a signal that the system has lost balance, not simply that something is damaged. The same structure can behave very differently depending on how it is used, supported, and regulated.

Recognizing that back or neck pain is complex is not discouraging but it is liberating. It shifts the question from "What is wrong with my back or neck?" to "Why did I get back or neck pain?". This shift opens the door to approaches that are more individualized, and more sustainable.

Before exploring biomechanics, anatomy, or therapeutic practices, it is important to accept this complexity. Without doing so, the search for simple answers can lead to disappointment. With it, we become ready to look deeper.

The following case studies explain this complexity in real lives. They reveal how similar findings can lead to relatively different outcomes and why understanding back or neck pain requires more than a single explanation.

# TWO CASES, TWO CHOICES

If back or neck pain were simple, similar findings would lead to similar outcomes. In practice, this rarely happens. Over the years, working with individuals seeking relief from pain, I have witnessed a striking pattern. People with comparable diagnoses, similar imaging reports, and even similar symptoms often travel very different paths. Their choices, circumstances, and the way their bodies respond, shapes the outcome far more than the diagnosis alone.

The following two case studies illustrate this clearly. They are not presented to judge medical decisions or promote a single approach, but to reveal how pain behaves when the human system is viewed beyond structure alone.

## The First Case: When Structure Was Addressed, But Pain Persisted

The first case involves a young individual who experienced persistent lower back pain in her late teens. An MRI scan revealed a disc herniation between the fourth and fifth lumbar vertebrae. The intervertebral disc, which normally acts as a flexible cushion between bones, had protruded beyond its usual boundary. This finding is commonly labeled as a slipped or herniated disc.

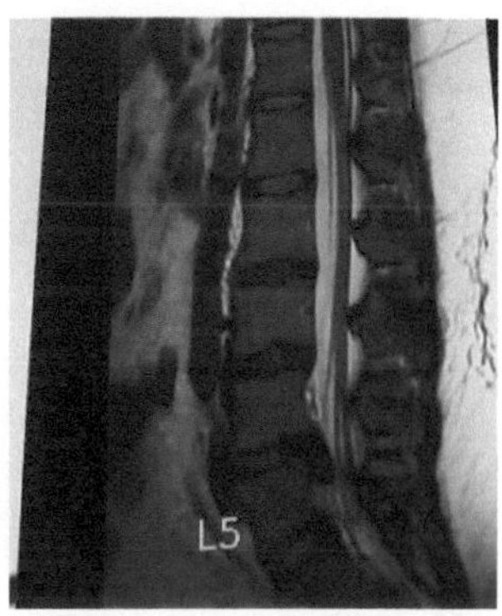

Based on the scan, surgery was recommended. The reasoning appeared logical. If the disc was pressing on surrounding structures and causing pain, removing it should provide relief. The procedure was performed, and the disc material was surgically addressed.

From a structural perspective, the problem seen on the image was corrected.

Yet, the pain persisted.

Years later, this individual came seeking Yoga therapy. What stood out immediately was not only the persistence of pain, but her age. She was just nineteen years old when the surgery was performed. Despite the intervention, she continued to experience discomfort, stiffness, and limitation.

This situation raises a difficult but a necessary question. If the structure that appeared problematic was surgically corrected, why did the pain remain?

The answer does not lie in questioning the intent of treatment, but in recognizing its limits. The surgery addressed what was visible. It did not address how her body moved, how muscles adapted around the surgical site, how fear and protection influenced posture, or how the nervous system continued to interpret threat.

The image had changed. The experience had not.

### The Second Case: When Structure Was Observed, But Not Removed

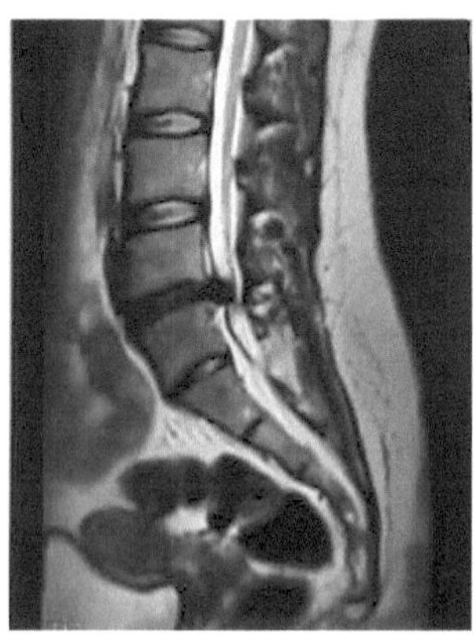

The second case involved another individual with back pain and an MRI report showing a disc bulge. Structurally, the findings were not dramatically different from the first case. However, the severity of symptoms was lower, and daily functioning was less restricted.

Once again, surgery was suggested as a possible option.

This time, a different choice was made.

Instead of proceeding with surgery, she chose to explore conservative management. Through carefully guided Yoga practices, she began working with her body rather than attempting to correct it structurally. The practices focused on restoring strength, improving flexibility, stabilizing the core, reducing unnecessary tension, developing more inner awareness and more importantly keeping herself calm as she moved and performed daily activities.

Over the past several years, she has managed her condition without surgical intervention. Pain has not disappeared permanently, but it has become understandable and manageable. When flare ups occur, returning to specific practices brings relief. Her body responds predictably, not fearfully.

What is important here is not the absence of pain, but the relationship with it. Her body retained its structural integrity and its capacity to adapt. She learned how to support it rather than override it.

## What These Two Cases Reveal?

These two cases are not exceptions. They reflect a broader pattern seen repeatedly in the world of physical pain. Structural findings alone do not determine the outcome. The same diagnosis can lead to very different experiences depending on how the body is supported, how movement is restored, how the nervous system is guided back towards safety and more importantly with what attitude the person wants to resolve the pain.

The first individual addressed pain by altering the structure. The second addressed pain by altering the function.

Neither of the paths guarantees success or failure. However, these cases highlight an essential truth. Pain does not arise from structure in isolation. It emerges from how the body organizes itself around structure over time.

> ***When pain is approached only through correction of what is seen, important contributors remain untouched. When pain is approached as a system-level experience, new possibilities to heal emerge.***

These stories are not meant to promote avoidance of medical intervention. Surgery has its place and can be life changing when clearly indicated. The purpose here is discernment. Understanding when structure truly requires intervention, and when the body needs support, awareness, and time.

The question is not which choice is right. The question is whether the choice is informed by a complete understanding of how pain works.

To answer that question, we must look more closely at the tools we rely on to define pain, especially imaging. This leads us to examine a crucial issue in modern healthcare, the assumption that what we see on a scan explains what a person feels.

# WHEN IMAGES DO NOT TELL THE WHOLE STORY

Modern technology has given us remarkable tools to look inside a human body. Among these, Magnetic Resonance Imaging or MRI occupies a central place in the diagnosis of spinal conditions. MRI scans provide detailed views of bones and soft tissues such as intervertebral discs, ligaments, and nerves. Because of this clarity, MRI findings are often treated as an authoritative explanation for pain.

Yet, when it comes to chronic back and neck pain, images do not always tell the whole story.

An MRI shows what the body looks like at a particular moment in time. It does not show how the body moves, how it distributes load, how it adapts to stress, or how the nervous system interprets signals. It captures structure, but not function. It records anatomy, but not lived experience.

This distinction becomes important when we examine research on the relationship between MRI findings and pain.

A systematic review of 33 studies involving 3,110 asymptomatic individuals found that disc degeneration was present in approximately 37 percent of 20-year-olds, increasing to 52 percent by age 30 and 68 percent by age 40[(1)]. Disc bulges were seen in about 30 to 50 percent of asymptomatic adults across these age groups. Disc protrusions occurred in roughly 29 to 33 percent. Annular tears were identified in about 19 to 22 percent of individuals between 20 and 40 years of age.

These findings challenge the assumption that structural abnormalities seen on MRI necessarily explain pain. Many degenerative changes appear to be part of normal aging rather than definitive evidence of a pain-generating pathology. This highlights a disconnect between what is visible on imaging and what is actually experienced by the person.

This leads to an unavoidable question.

If many healthy people show these abnormalities without pain, can we assume the similar abnormalities are the direct cause of pain in those who are suffering?

The implications are significant. When MRI findings are treated as definitive explanations, decisions may be driven more by images than by the lived experience of the patient. This can lead to unnecessary or invasive interventions without addressing the factors that truly sustain pain.

This does not mean MRI scans are useless. They are essential in cases involving trauma, progressive neurological deficits, infection, or serious structural compromise. The concern arises when imaging becomes the primary lens through which pain is understood, rather than one component of a broader assessment.

When patients are told that their pain exists because something is wrong or damaged in their spine, fear often follows. Movement begins to feel dangerous. The body becomes guarded. Muscles tighten, breathing changes, and the nervous system shifts into vigilance. These protective responses can amplify pain, even when the structural findings are stable or benign.

What is often missing is a holistic approach.

Pain does not exist in isolation from habitual movements, lifestyle, emotional state, conditioning, and adaptive behavior. Two people with identical MRI findings may experience pain very differently depending on how their bodies move, how their muscles support them, how their nervous systems regulate threat, and how they interpret discomfort.

The findings from Dr. Brinjikji's study[1] strongly support a more holistic approach to back pain. Such an approach does not dismiss structural information, but places it within a wider context that includes physical, psychological, and environmental factors.

Yoga therapy works within this broader framework. It emphasizes understanding the person rather than treating the image. Practices are tailored, adjusted through feedback, and oriented toward restoring balance rather than correcting structure alone. Movement, breath, posture, mindset, and awareness influence how the body adapts and how pain is perceived.

This stands in contrast to decisions made solely on the basis of MRI results, which may not correlate with the actual experience of pain.

Images show us what exists. They do not explain how the body arrived there, or how it will respond in the future. To understand pain fully, we must look beyond what is visible and listen to the intelligence of the living system.

# ORGANIC AND FUNCTIONAL CAUSES OF PHYSICAL PAIN

As we move toward a deeper understanding of physical pain, it becomes essential to distinguish between different kinds of causes. Not all pain arises in the same way, and not all pain should be approached with the same strategy. One of the most helpful ways to clarify this is by recognizing the difference between organic and functional causes of pain. This understanding is crucial to understand why MRI cannot reveal everything.

This distinction does not create a hierarchy. One is not more real than the other. Both are valid. However, they require very different forms of attention and response.

Organic causes refer to physical changes or abnormalities within the body that can be identified through medical examination, imaging, or laboratory tests. These causes involve structural disruption or pathological processes that directly affect tissues.

Examples of organic causes include tumors that exert pressure on the spine or nerves, infections such as tuberculosis, osteomyelitis or discitis that involve inflammation of bone or disc tissue, and major injuries resulting from accidents or severe falls that cause fractures, significant disc damage, or instability. Other organic causes include pronounced anatomical changes in the spine such as spinal stenosis, advanced osteoarthritis, or severe scoliosis.

When pain arises from organic causes, medical intervention is often necessary and sometimes urgent. In such cases, treatments may include medication, injections, surgical procedures, or emergency care. These conditions are usually well defined, and delaying appropriate medical treatment can lead to serious complications.

Yoga does not replace medical care in these situations. Its role, when appropriate, is supportive and rehabilitative rather than primary.

Functional causes of pain, in contrast, do not arise from visible structural damage or disease. Instead, they emerge from how the body is used, conditioned, stressed, and adapted over time. These causes are often invisible on imaging, yet they account for a large proportion of chronic pain experienced by people today.

Functional causes include sedentary lifestyles, inadequate physical activity, repetitive strain, and movement patterns that place sustained stress on certain parts of the body. Chronic poor posture while sitting, standing, walking, running or working can gradually overload muscles and joints, leading to pain that develops slowly and persists.

Psychological stress also plays a significant role. Stress frequently manifests as increased muscle tension, particularly in the back, neck, and shoulders. When this tension becomes habitual, it alters posture, breathing, and nervous system regulation, contributing to pain. We shall understand about this in detail in the coming chapters.

Excess body weight places additional mechanical load on the spine, especially the lower back. Poor nutrition can further weaken muscles and bones, reducing their ability to support the body effectively.

What makes functional causes particularly important is that they are often preventable and manageable. They respond well to changes in lifestyle, movement, awareness, and self-care.

Understanding whether pain is primarily organic or functional is not about labeling. It is about choosing the right path of care.

# THE SCALE OF THE PROBLEM: BACK AND NECK PAIN IN NUMBERS

Before we move into the mechanics of movement, it is important to pause and appreciate the scale of the problem we are addressing. Back and neck pain are not marginal conditions. They are among the most widespread and persistent sources of physical suffering across the world. Those who are not interested in statistics can skip this chapter and move on to the next one.

Back pain and Neck pain affects millions globally and has emerged as one of the leading causes of disability. The Global Burden of Disease study published in *The Lancet* identifies low back pain and neck pain as the largest contributor to years lived with disability worldwide, highlighting its profound impact on quality of life, productivity, and overall well-being effecting diverse age groups and regions[(2)(3)].

Research further suggests that approximately 70 to 80 percent of individuals will experience low back pain at some point in their lives, underscoring its near-universal occurrence[(4)(5)]. Its prevalence increases with age and remains high from middle age onward, continuing to be a major contributor to disability across populations[(4)]. Neck pain, although it can occur at any stage of life, it is found to be more common during midlife and often follows a recurrent course rather than a single acute episode[(6)]. While many episodes improve, a meaningful proportion of individuals develop persistent symptoms that diminish quality of life and increase the use of healthcare[(6)]. This widespread occurrence underscores the importance of prevention, ergonomic awareness, and holistic management.

The economic consequences are equally significant. In the United States alone, musculoskeletal conditions, including back pain, account for over 260 million lost workdays annually, reflecting substantial effects on productivity and healthcare utilization[7]. When adjusted for inflation, the current burden is likely far greater. These costs arise not only from medical care, but also from lost wages and reduced functional capacity. Collectively, these findings emphasize the need for preventive strategies and comprehensive approaches that address behavioural and lifestyle factors alongside structural considerations.

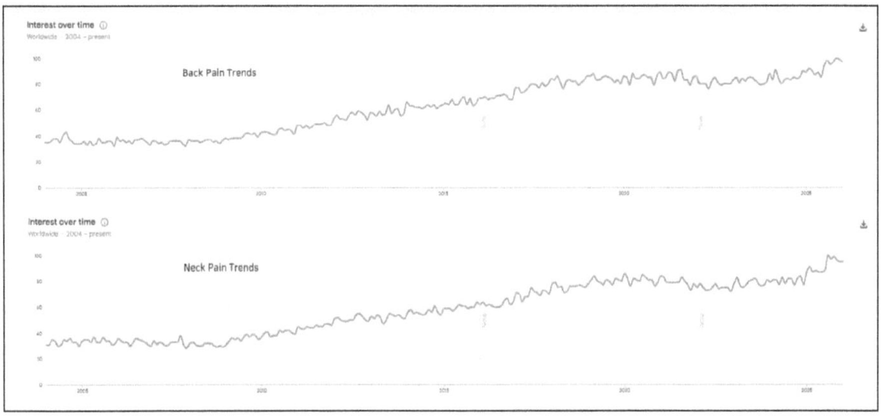


**FIGURE 1:** Google search trends for back pain and Neck Pain search

The digital age allows people to seek instant information on health concerns, and back and neck pain are no exceptions. Worldwide Google Trends data Figure 1 shows consistently high and rising search volumes for back and neck pain, reflecting the global concern surrounding these conditions. While the internet offers access to diverse perspectives and remedies, it also requires discernment to distinguish reliable information from the questionable. The sheer volume of searches reveals both the prevalence of pain and the urgency with which people seek relief.

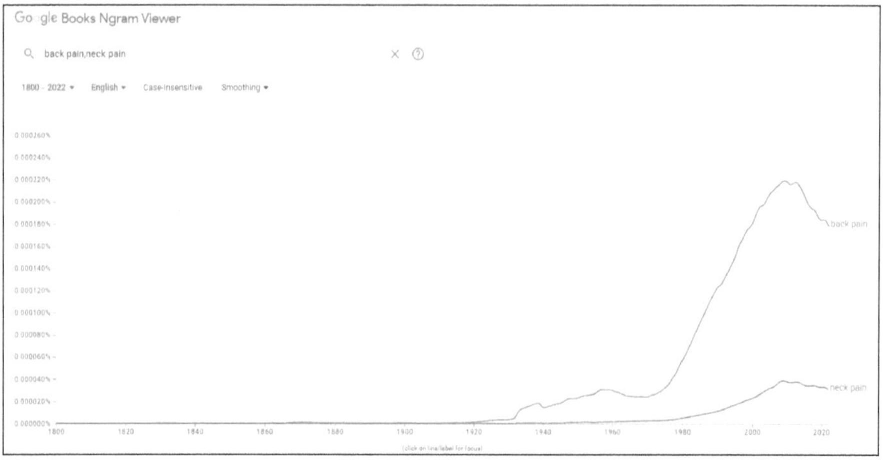


**FIGURE 2:** Google books Nrgam viewer on back pain

The Google Books Ngram Viewer, a tool that tracks the frequency of phrases published in books over time, shows a notable increase in discussions about back pain and neck pain starting in the 1990s as shown in Figure 2. This increase in literary attention suggests a rising awareness and prevalence of back and neck issues among the general population during this period. It reflects broader societal concerns, perhaps prompted by emerging health trends and changes in daily activities due to technological advancements.

The 1990s marked the beginning of the IT revolution, characterized by the rapid expansion of computer-based jobs and digital communication tools. This period led to the proliferation of desk jobs that require long hours in front of computer screens. Such sedentary job roles drastically reduced daily physical activity for many workers, confining them to their desks for the majority of the workday.

A sedentary lifestyle is now widely recognized as a risk factor for spinal discomfort. Prolonged sitting, especially with poor posture, increases stress on spinal discs and supporting tissues, often leading to chronic pain[(4)]. The alignment between rising literature and technological change suggests that modern work habits have played a meaningful role in this growing concern. As the digital era continues to evolve, discussions around spinal health remain essential. Promoting movement, improving ergonomics, and taking regular breaks are becoming increasingly important preventive measures.

This observation raises an important question. If back and neck pain affect such a large proportion of the population across cultures and professions, why do conventional approaches so often fall short?

Part of the answer may lie in how pain is conceptualized. When pain is viewed primarily as a structural defect to be corrected, important dimensions are overlooked. Movement patterns, nervous system regulation, emotional stress, habitual posture, and adaptive behavior all influence how pain develops and persists.

Yoga offers a framework that addresses these dimensions together[(8)]. By working simultaneously with the body, breath, and awareness, Yoga engages aspects of pain that remain invisible in statistics and imaging reports. As more individuals turn toward integrative approaches, the possibility of reducing the long-term burden of back and neck pain becomes not only hopeful, but necessary.

Understanding the scale of the problem prepares us for the next step. To address pain meaningfully, we must understand how the body responds to forces, adapts to habits, and organizes itself in daily life.

But before we get there, let us ask a deeper question.

Why does the back or neck, more than many other parts of the body, so often become the site where pain manifests?

# WHY THE SPINE, ESPECIALLY THE BACK AND NECK, IS PARTICULARLY VULNERABLE?

One of the most common questions that arises when discussing physical pain is why the spine is so frequently affected. Why do discomfort and dysfunction appear so often in the back and neck rather than in the arms, the legs, or other parts of the body with equal frequency? The answer lies in a combination of anatomy, biomechanics, and human evolution.

The human spine is a marvel of natural engineering. It provides both stability and flexibility, allowing us to bend, twist, reach, lift, rotate, and orient ourselves in space. These capabilities are essential for daily life. Yet, the very versatility that makes the spine so functional, also makes it vulnerable when demand exceed support.

A key factor in this vulnerability is our evolution from being four-legged animals, to walk on two legs. This shift carries profound implications for spinal health, affecting both the lower back and the neck.

In an upright posture, the spine must support the weight of the head, torso, and upper limbs while balancing this load over a relatively small base formed by the feet. Gravity acts continuously on this vertical structure, requiring subtle and constant muscular adjustments to maintain balance. Over time, especially when muscles are under-conditioned or movement patterns become inefficient, these adjustments can lead to fatigue and strain.

The lumbar spine carries a particularly heavy burden. It supports much of the body's weight and acts as a central pivot for movement. Its natural curvature aids shock absorption but also increases mechanical load. When combined with prolonged sitting, poor posture, or repetitive strain, this region becomes especially susceptible to discomfort.

The cervical spine faces a different but equally demanding role. The human head weighs approximately four to five kilograms, and when it is well balanced over the shoulders, the effort required to support it is minimal. However, even a slight forward shift dramatically increases the mechanical load on the neck[9]. What begins as a small postural change can translate into significant muscular effort and joint stress.

Modern lifestyles intensify this challenge. Hours spent looking at screens, working on computers, or using mobile devices encourage the head to drift forward. The muscles of the neck and upper back must then work continuously to prevent further collapse. Over time, this sustained effort leads to fatigue, tightness, and altered movement patterns. What begins as adaptation gradually becomes habit, and habit eventually becomes discomfort.

In contrast, quadrupeds distribute body weight across four limbs, with the head supported more in line with the spine rather than balanced vertically above it. This arrangement reduces the load on any single spinal segment. Humans, by comparison, carry weight directly downward through the spine, increasing stress on discs and joints throughout the column.

Seen in this light, back and neck pain are rarely isolated failures. They are signals from a structure performing an inherently demanding task under the constant influence of gravity.

Understanding this changes our perspective. Instead of viewing pain as evidence that something has gone wrong, we begin to see it as communication from a system adapting to the way it is being used.

To understand this process more clearly, we must now turn our attention to biomechanics. By examining how forces act on the body and how movement distributes load, we begin to see why certain patterns lead to pain and how those patterns can be transformed.

PART II

# UNDERSTANDING THE BODY AS A LIVING SYSTEM

# UNDERSTANDING BIOMECHANICS THROUGH SIMPLE ANALOGIES

To understand back pain, neck pain and the biomechanics behind spinal health, we often need a way to make invisible forces visible. Biomechanics can sound technical, but at its heart it is simply the study of how forces act on the body and how the body responds to those forces.

An analogy that illustrates how forces travel through the spine is that of a train collision.

Imagine two trains travelling toward each other and colliding head-on. The moment they crash, an enormous force is generated at the point of impact. But that force does not remain only at the front. It travels through the entire length of both trains. Every coach, every link in the train experiences that transmitted force.

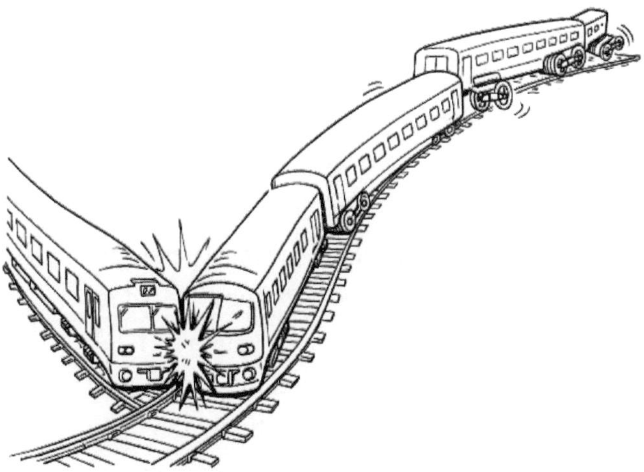

What is interesting is that not every part of the train suffers damage in the same way. The front coaches may remain on the track because they are directly engaged and designed to meet force. But coaches further back, which are not directly at the point of impact, might derail or even get ripped off the track. This happens because the force gets distributed through the train, and the weakest link in that chain is the one that fails first. It is not always the part that was closest to the crash but it is the part that was least able to handle the forces coming through it.

> ***This is the key principle the analogy reveals. When force travels through a connected system, damage often appears where the system is the weakest, and not necessarily where the force originates.***

Now let us bring this back to the human body.

Your entire body is also a connected system. It is made of many segments stacked one above another, from the neck down to the feet. Each vertebral segment of your spine, each segment of your body between two joints can be thought of as one coach of the train. No single segment works alone. Each segment participates in distributing load and supporting movement of the body. Just as force travels through all the coaches of a train during a collision, forces travel through all segments of the body during daily life.

The most important difference is that, unlike a train collision which is rare, the major force acting on our body is present every moment of our lives.

That force is gravity.

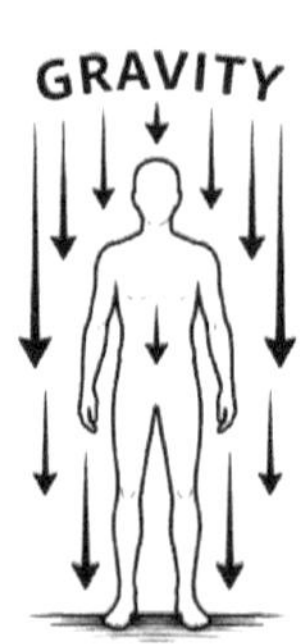


Gravity is constantly pulling us downward. It is so familiar that we rarely notice it, yet it is the most persistent force the body must negotiate. Every posture we adopt and every movement we perform happens within its field. Standing, sitting, bending, walking, running, lifting, and even lying down are shaped by how effectively the body manages gravity.

In the train analogy, the force is sudden and dramatic. In the human body, gravity is continuous and subtle. Yet, because it acts day after day, year after year, its cumulative effect is profound. The body must continuously distribute this force through the spine, pelvis, legs, and feet. When the system is well organized, gravity flows through it smoothly. Muscles work just enough to maintain support, joints share load efficiently, and movement feels relatively effortless.

Once this organization is disturbed, gravity no longer distributes forces evenly and stress begins to accumulate in specific regions.

This brings us back to the idea of the weak link.

Just as the weakest coach derails first, the segment of the body least prepared to handle load often becomes the site where pain appears. For many people this is the lower back, which carries significant weight and participates in almost every movement. For others it may be the neck, the mid-back, the hips, or the knees. The location varies, but the principle remains unchanged.

> ***Pain often appears where the system is least able to manage the forces travelling through it.***

This understanding also explains why pain is not always located at the root of the problem. An imbalance in one region quietly forces another region to compensate. Over time, the compensating area becomes overloaded, and the person experiences pain there. It is natural to assume that the painful area is the primary issue, but this assumption can be misleading.

To understand this more deeply, we must look at how the body manages balance, because balance determines how gravity moves through us. A key concept here is the center of gravity. Many imagine it as a fixed point somewhere within the torso, but in reality it is constantly shifting. Every change in posture and every movement alters its position.

Consider the simple act of standing. When weight is distributed evenly through both feet, the center of gravity remains relatively stable. The spine stacks naturally, and the muscles do not need to overwork.

But if a person habitually shifts weight onto one side, the center moves away from the midline. The body must immediately compensate to prevent falling. The pelvis adjusts, the spine reorganizes, and muscles throughout the body change their tone. These compensations may be subtle, yet when repeated daily they become habitual patterns.

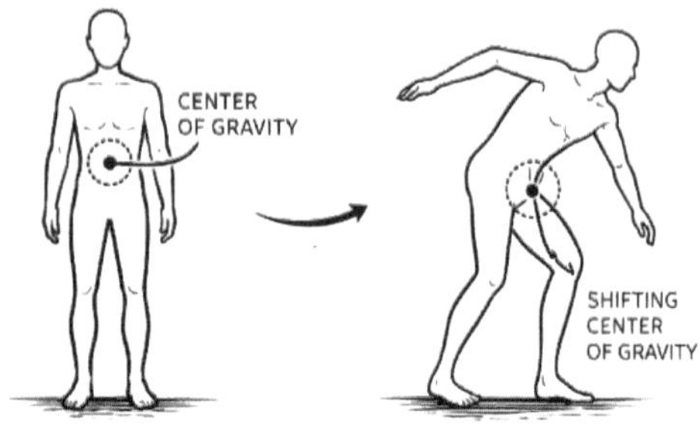


Now consider leaning forward to pick something up. As the torso moves forward, the center of gravity shifts forward. If this shift is managed well, the hips, legs, and spine share the load. If it is not, a single region, often the lower back or the neck, absorbs disproportionate stress.

Running provides another illustration. With each stride, the body briefly moves beyond its base of support and then regains balance. Efficient movement allows forces to pass smoothly through the system. Inefficient patterns transmit excessive impact upward into the spine.

These examples reveal an important insight: Pain is not always about how heavy the load is. It is often about how well the body manages shifting load.

Gravity also does not act purely downward. When posture is distorted, it creates rotational and shearing forces within the body. A tilted pelvis or a habitually forward head changes how gravity passes through the spine. Muscles must resist these deviations continuously, and over time this resistance leads to fatigue, tightness, and discomfort.

Even stillness can become demanding. Prolonged sitting with poor alignment forces the body to resist gravity without the relief that movement provides. Muscles remain engaged, joints remain compressed, and circulation is reduced. What appears to be rest quietly becomes another form of strain.

The body responds intelligently to these demands. It tightens where stability is required and relaxes where it can. But when imbalanced postures or movements are repeated day after day, these responses become habits. The body learns to hold itself in ways that manage gravity under those conditions, even when those conditions are not ideal.

This is why pain often develops gradually rather than suddenly. There may be no single injury, only the slow accumulation of stress as gravity is managed inefficiently over time. Eventually, the weakest link begins to signal distress.

Understanding gravity and balance also transforms how we think about posture correction. Simply trying to sit or stand straight often increases tension because it ignores the deeper issue of balance. True postural change occurs when the body learns to distribute force more efficiently. When balance improves, posture reorganizes naturally.

This perspective invites compassion rather than blame. The body has been doing its best to manage gravity under the conditions it was given. Healing begins not by forcing the body into ideal positions, but by teaching it better ways to balance and distribute force.

Once we understand this, an important shift occurs. Instead of asking, where is the pain? we begin to ask, how is force travelling through the body, and why is it concentrating here?

That question becomes the foundation for everything that follows in this book.

It also leads us to a deeper inquiry. How does the body decide where to adapt? How does it learn what to strengthen and what to let go? To answer that, we must look beyond mechanics and begin to understand the intelligence inherent in the human body itself.

# THE HUMAN BODY IS NOT A MACHINE

To understand how back and neck pain develop over time, it is helpful to compare the human body with mechanical systems. This comparison is useful not because the body is a machine, but because certain mechanical principles make patterns of use and misuse easier to understand. At the same time, it is important to recognize where the comparison ends, because the human body is far more adaptive and intelligent than any machine we build.

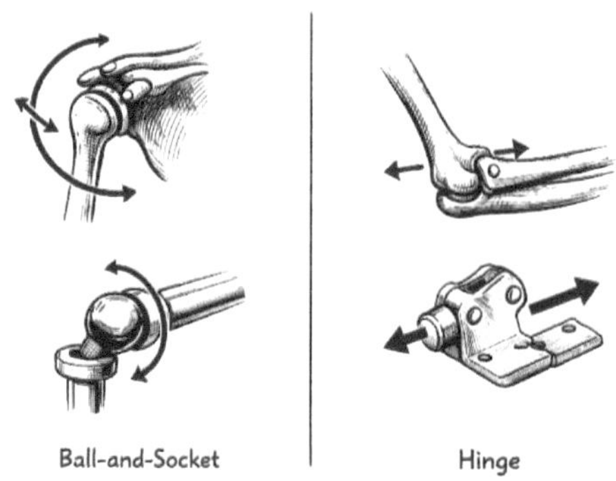


Many joints in the human body resemble mechanical designs. The shoulders and hips function much like ball-and-socket mechanisms, allowing movement in multiple directions. This design supports activities that require reaching, turning, and rotation. The knees, elbows, and wrists function more like hinges, permitting movement primarily in one plane. This structure allows efficient bending and straightening, which is essential for walking, lifting, and daily tasks.

These parallels help us understand that the human body, like any well-designed mechanical system, is built to perform specific functions. When joints are used in ways that respect their design, movement feels smooth and effortless. When they are used repeatedly in distorted or excessive ways, strain begins to appear.

Mechanical systems also respond predictably to patterns of use. Consider a car that is driven two thousand kilometers every day. Even if it is well built, such intense usage would quickly lead to wear and tear. Regular servicing would become necessary, and without it, parts would fail prematurely. On the other hand, consider a car that remains unused in a garage for two years. Even with minimal use, the engine may seize, fluids may degrade, components may deteriorate, and the car may fail to start when the ignition is turned. Lack of use can be just as damaging as overuse.

The human body responds in a remarkably similar way.

When certain muscles, joints, or movement patterns are overused without adequate recovery, they become strained. Repetitive stress accumulates, and tissues lose their capacity to adapt. This often shows up as chronic back or neck pain, particularly in people whose work or exercise routines repeatedly load the same regions of the body.

At the same time, underuse has its own consequences. When muscles and joints are not used regularly, they weaken and stiffen. Range of motion reduces, coordination declines, and the body becomes less prepared to handle sudden demands. This is why people who are mostly sedentary often experience pain when they perform even simple physical tasks. The system has not been trained to manage the forces involved.

Modern lifestyles often push us towards one of these two extremes. On one end, there is an emphasis on high-intensity activity, where the idea that more is better dominates. Bodies are pushed hard with little regard for recovery or balance. On the other end, many people spend long hours sitting, especially in front of screens, with minimal movement throughout the day. Both extremes disrupt the body's natural rhythm of use and rest.

What these patterns reveal is that the body learns from how it is treated. Repetition shapes structure and function. Movements that are performed frequently become easier and more efficient. Movements that are avoided become difficult and uncomfortable. This learning process is not conscious.

It happens automatically, driven by the body's need to function efficiently under the conditions it experiences most often.

This is where the comparison with machines begins to fall short.

Machines do not heal themselves. They do not reorganize based on experience. They require external intervention to repair damage. The human body, by contrast, has an inherent capacity to heal, adapt, and improve when given appropriate conditions. Muscles strengthen in response to use. Bones become denser when loaded appropriately. Movement patterns refine themselves through practice.

Yoga provides a clear example of this adaptive process. Through varied postures and movements, Yoga engages different parts of the body in a balanced way. No single joint or muscle group is overworked or ignored. The practice encourages awareness, allowing practitioners to recognize the difference between healthy effort and harmful strain. Over time, the body learns new patterns of movement and postures that are more sustainable.

This learning is not about forcing the body into ideal shapes. It is about offering experiences that the body can integrate. When movement is balanced and mindful, the body updates its internal maps. Coordination improves and tension reduces. Pain often diminishes without aggressive intervention.

Understanding the body in this way changes our approach to healing. Instead of treating pain as a mechanical failure that must be fixed, we begin to see it as feedback from a system that has adapted to certain patterns. Those patterns can be changed, not through force, but through intelligent use of the body.

Ultimately, we can conclude that, the human body is not a machine, but like a well-designed system, it responds predictably to how it is used. When used in balance, the body thrives. When it is overused or underused, body disfunctions. Recognizing this principle prepares us to explore the deeper intelligence that governs adaptation and healing, which is the focus of the next chapter.

# BODY INTELLIGENCE, TENSEGRITY, AND THE CHAIN REACTION OF IMBALANCE

To understand pain, healing, and long-term health, we must begin with a fundamental principle. The body is not passive. It is intelligent. This intelligence is not located in one organ or system. It is present throughout the body, expressed through the constant ability to sense, adapt, and reorganize in response to how we live.

This inherent capacity is often referred to as body intelligence. It is the reason muscles grow stronger when they are used, bones become denser when they are loaded, and coordination improves with practice. It is also the reason muscles weaken when they are not used, joints stiffen with immobility, and discomfort emerges when the system loses balance.

The body does not make these changes out of error but it makes them due to demand. It allocates resources according to demand. What is used is supported. What is not used is gradually deprioritized. This principle can be observed easily in daily life. A person who writes predominantly with one hand develops greater strength and control in that hand over time. The adaptation is not conscious. The body simply responds to repeated demand.

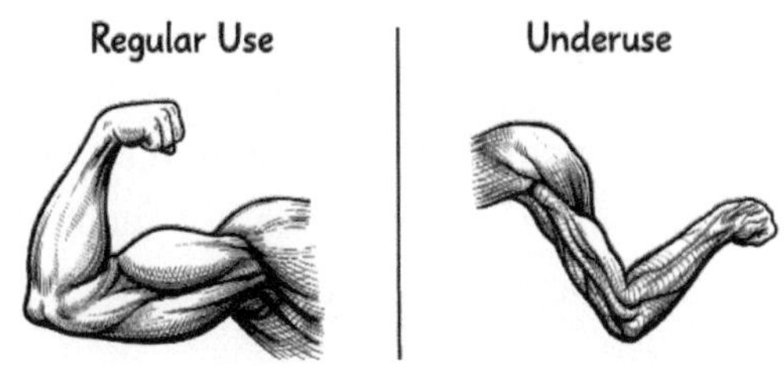


The same intelligence governs the entire musculoskeletal system. When muscles and joints are used regularly and appropriately, they remain responsive and resilient. When they are underused, the body reduces investment in them. Muscle fibers shrink, neural connections weaken, and joint nourishment decreases. This process is often described medically as disuse atrophy, but it is better understood as the body's intelligent response to inactivity.

A clear example of this process appears during immobilization after injury. When a limb is placed in a cast, movement is restricted to allow healing. Once the cast is removed, several changes are immediately noticeable. The muscles appear smaller, the joint feels stiff, and strength is reduced.

None of this is accidental. During immobilization, the body recognizes that the area is not being used and conserves energy accordingly. From the body's perspective, this is efficient. From the individual's perspective, it can feel alarming.

What matters is not that this change occurs, but how it is addressed afterward. When movement is reintroduced gradually and intelligently, the body adapts again. Muscles regain strength, joints regain mobility, and coordination returns. The body updates its internal understanding of what is required. This adaptive intelligence works in both directions.

In modern life, many individuals experience a form of immobilization without injury. Long hours of sitting, limited variation in posture, and reduced physical activity signal to the body that large portions of the system are no longer needed. Over time, muscles that support posture weaken, joints lose range of motion, and the nervous system becomes less confident in movement.

When movement is suddenly demanded after prolonged inactivity, pain often appears. This pain is not necessarily evidence of damage. It is frequently a signal that the system is unprepared for the demand being placed upon it.

At this point, it becomes important to recognize another essential feature of the body. The body does not function as a collection of independent parts. It functions as a connected system in which each region influences the others.

One concept that helps explain this interconnectedness is tensegrity, short for tensional integrity. Though the word may sound technical, the idea behind it is simple and deeply relevant to how the human body maintains its structure.

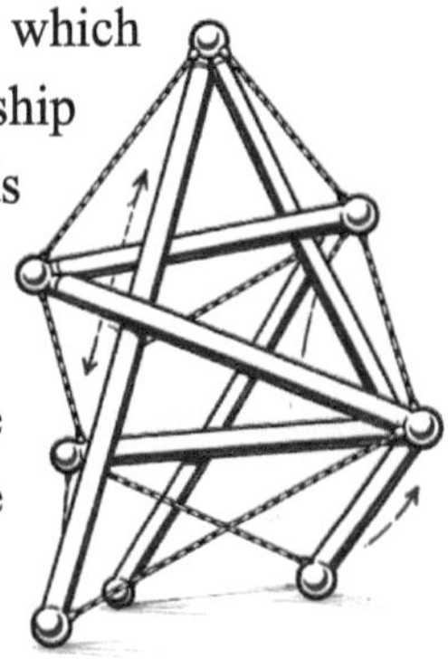

Tensegrity describes a type of structure in which stability is achieved through a balanced relationship between tension and compression. Imagine rigid rods suspended within a network of flexible cables. The rods provide form, while the cables maintain continuous tension. The structure holds its shape not because the rods are fixed together, but because tension is distributed evenly throughout the system. If tension changes in one cable, the entire structure adjusts.

The human body operates in a remarkably similar way. Bones provide shape and support, while muscles, and connective tissues create continuous tension that holds the structure together. Stability does not arise from bones stacking perfectly on top of one another. It arises from the balanced tension of the soft tissues that keep those bones in relationship.

This perspective changes how we understand posture. Posture is often thought of as a position that must be held or corrected. From the perspective of tensegrity, posture is a dynamic expression of how tension is distributed throughout the body. When tension is balanced, posture feels stable without effort. When tension becomes uneven, posture begins to distort, even if a person attempts to sit or stand correctly.

One of the most important implications of this model is that local problems rarely remain local. Because the body is a connected tensional system, changes in one area influence many others. A restriction, weakness, or habitual pattern in one region alters the distribution of tension across the entire structure. The body then compensates to maintain the balance.

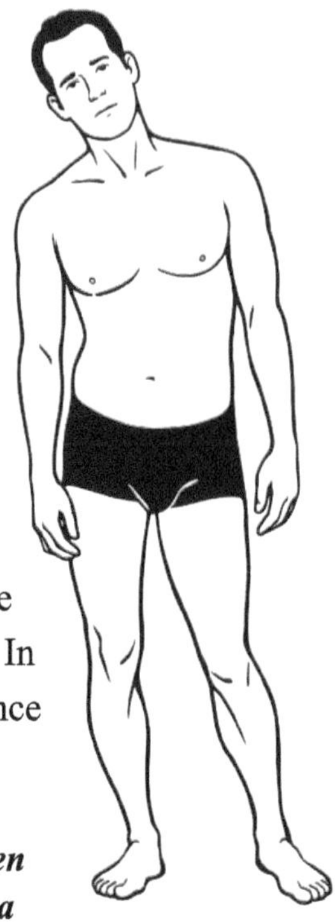

Consider a common habit such as standing with most of the body weight shifted onto one leg. This may feel natural, especially if it has been done unconsciously for years. Yet this simple shift sets off a cascade of adjustments. The pelvis tilts, the spine reorganizes to keep the head upright, the rib cage shifts, and the neck adapts in response to changes below.

Over time, muscles on one side of the neck may become overworked while others become lengthened and less active. Pain may appear in the neck, leading the person to believe that the neck is the primary problem. In reality, the neck is responding intelligently to imbalance elsewhere.

> ***This illustrates an important principle. Pain often appears at the weakest link in the chain, the area that has been compensating the longest or working the hardest to maintain overall stability.***

The tensegrity model helps explain why treating only the painful area often provides temporary relief. Addressing one tight muscle or restricted joint without restoring balance to the larger system leaves the underlying pattern unchanged. The body naturally returns to familiar compensation.

It also clarifies why posture cannot be corrected through force. Attempting to hold the body in an ideal position without redistributing tension increases strain. The system resists because the effort required to maintain that position is not shared evenly. True postural change occurs when the distribution of tension throughout the body changes.

This change happens gradually. As awareness improves and movement becomes more balanced, tissues that were overworking begin to release, while underused areas begin to engage. Muscles reorganize, coordination improves, and the body finds a new equilibrium. Posture improves not because it is imposed, but because it becomes the easiest way for the body to organize itself.

Understanding tensegrity also reframes how we view stability. Stability does not mean stiffness. A stiff structure cannot adapt to force. A well-balanced structure absorbs and redistributes force efficiently. In the human body, this translates to resilience, the ability to respond to load and movement without unnecessary strain.

Practices such as Yoga naturally supports this form of organization. By encouraging balanced strength, mobility, and awareness, they help distribute effort more evenly across the body. Movements are approached with attention rather than force, allowing the system to adjust without shock.

When we understand body intelligence and interconnectedness together, pain begins to make sense. It is no longer seen as a mysterious failure of one part of the body. More often, it is a signal that balance has been lost somewhere in the system.

Restoring that balance does not mean fixing a single area. It means allowing the whole structure to reorganize itself. And when it does, the chain reaction of imbalance gradually gives way to a chain reaction of support.

# THE SPINE AS A LIVING STRUCTURE

In the previous chapters, we explored how physical pain develops through adaptation rather than damage alone. By now, it should be clear that pain is rarely the result of a single faulty structure. It is more often the outcome of how the body has been used, held, and protected over time.

With this perspective established, we can now look at some anatomy.

Anatomy is often introduced early in discussions on pain, sometimes before any context is provided. When that happens, structures can appear fragile or defective, and normal variations can feel threatening. This book has intentionally placed anatomy here after introducing the ideas of adaptation, learning, and system-wide response have been understood.

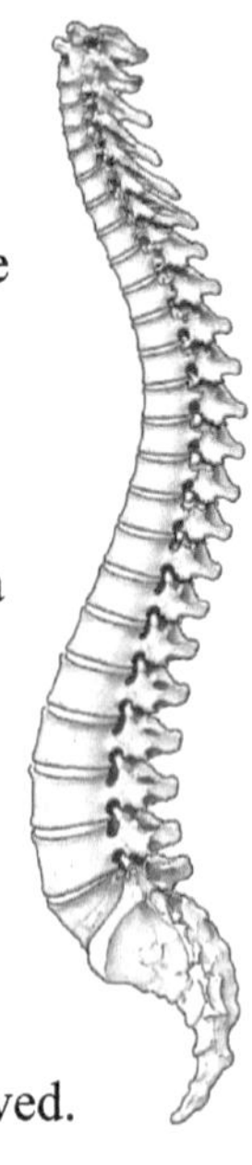

The chapters that follow are not meant to teach diagnosis or interpretation of scans. They are meant to offer just enough anatomical clarity to support understanding. Anatomy here serves as a map, and not as a verdict.

Let us begin with the human spine.

When people think of the spine, they often imagine it as a rigid column of bones stacked one over the other. This image is misleading. The spine is not a fixed structure designed only to hold the body upright. It is a living, adaptive system meant to move, respond, and reorganize continuously.

One of the first misconceptions to clear is the idea that a healthy spine is straight. The human spine is naturally curved.

From the side, it forms a gentle double S shape. These curves are not flaws or deviations. They are essential to how the spine functions. They help distribute load, absorb shock, and allow the body to remain resilient during movement.

Each curve serves a purpose. They allow the spine to respond to gravity instead of resisting it. When these curves are present and balanced, movement feels lighter and more stable. When they are exaggerated or flattened, strain begins to accumulate.

The spine is also not a single unit. It is a sequence of segments, each capable of small movements. These small movements add up to flexibility and balance. The health of the spine depends not on how rigid it is, but on how well these segments cooperate.

A rigid spine may appear strong, but rigidity is not strength. Rigidity limits the spine's ability to absorb force and instead transfers stress to specific points. Over time, this can lead to discomfort.

A healthy spine, by contrast, is stable without being stiff. It supports the body while remaining responsive. This balance between stability and mobility allows the spine to function as a living structure rather than a mechanical rod.

Another important aspect of the spine is its relationship with gravity. The spine is constantly organizing itself in response to gravity, whether we are standing, sitting, or lying down.

When posture is balanced, gravity flows through the body efficiently. Muscles work minimally, and breathing remains free. When posture is distorted, muscles tighten to compensate. Over time, this compensation leads to fatigue and discomfort.

This is why posture cannot be reduced to holding oneself upright. Forced uprightness often increases tension rather than improving alignment. True alignment arises when the spine is allowed to stack itself naturally in response to gravity, supported by balanced muscular engagement rather than effort.

The spine is also shaped by how we use the body each day. Repeated postures, habitual movements, and prolonged positions slowly influence its resting state. This does not happen overnight. It happens gradually, as the body adapts to what it is asked to do most often.

In this sense, the spine is a record of lived experience. Structural changes in the spine are often not signs of damage, but signs of adaptation.

> ***Understanding the spine as a living structure change how we approach pain. Pain does not necessarily mean something is broken. It often means that the spine has adapted to conditions that no longer serve it well.***

This perspective also helps reduce fear. When the spine is seen as fragile, people become hesitant to move. When it is seen as living and adaptable, movement becomes part of healing rather than something to be avoided.

The spine is designed to move, respond, and change. It is not meant to be shielded from daily use, but rather supported through intelligent use. When we respect its living nature, we begin to work with the body rather than against it.

This understanding lays the foundation for everything that follows. To understand pain, posture, and healing, we must first recognize that the spine is not a static structure to be fixed, but a living system capable of learning, adapting, and restoring balance over time.

# DISCS, JOINTS, AND MOVEMENT BETWEEN THE BONES

When people hear terms such as disc bulge, disc degeneration, or slipped disc, fear often follows immediately. Discs are often spoken about as though they are fragile structures that can suddenly fail. To understand back and neck pain clearly, it is important to look at what discs and joints actually are, and how they are meant to function.

Between each pair of vertebrae lies an intervertebral disc. These discs are not solid blocks. They are living, flexible structures designed to allow movement and absorb load. A disc deforms under pressure and returns to shape when the pressure is released. This adaptability is what allows the spine to bend, twist, and respond to everyday demands.

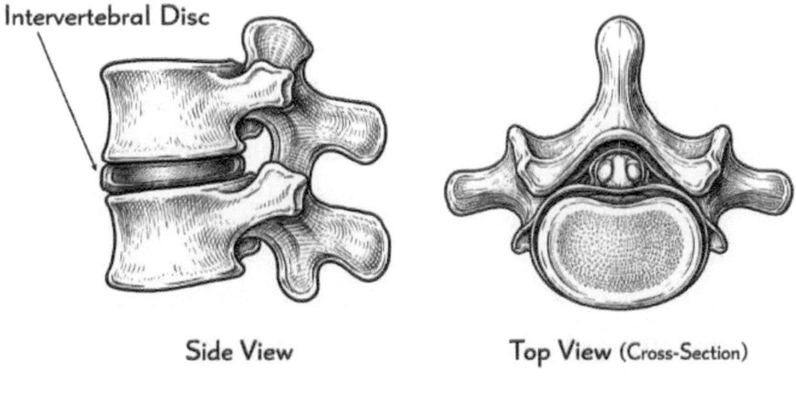


Discs do not work in isolation. They function together with the small joints behind the spine and the surrounding support system. Movement between the bones is shared. When this sharing happens well, stress is distributed evenly instead of concentrating in one place.

A common misconception is that discs remain healthy through rest. In reality, discs depend on movement to remain healthy. Because they have very limited direct blood supply, they receive nourishment through gentle compression and release. Movement allows fluid to move in and out, delivering nutrients and clearing waste.

When movement is reduced, this process is affected. Prolonged sitting, immobility, or fear-based avoidance of movement deprives the discs of nourishment. Over time, they may lose hydration and resilience. What is often labeled as degeneration is frequently the result of reduced movement rather than damage.

This is why complete rest rarely resolves disc-related pain. Short periods of rest may ease acute discomfort, but prolonged inactivity often increases stiffness and sensitivity. The spine is designed to be used constantly.

It is also important to recognize that discs naturally change with age. Just as skin loses elasticity over time, discs undergo gradual transformation. These changes are normal and do not automatically lead to pain. Many people live active, pain-free lives with disc changes visible on imaging.

Pain is influenced less by shape of the disc and more by how the spine is being used. When movement is uneven and certain segments carry more load than others, discs are subjected to abnormal forces. The disc then becomes a messenger rather than the root cause.

The joints between the vertebrae guide and regulate movement. When the movement is free and symmetrical, the spine remains adaptable. When it becomes restricted, movement is forced into fewer segments, and those segments begin to carry more load than they were meant to. This is why disc issues often appear at specific levels instead of throughout the spine. The problem is rarely that the disc itself is weak, but rather that the surrounding system has lost its balance.

Understanding this, shifts attention away from blaming the disc. Instead of asking what is wrong with a particular disc, we begin to ask how movement is being distributed through the spine.

With this foundation, it becomes easier to understand some of the common changes that are often described in spinal discs. These terms frequently appear in imaging reports and medical conversations, and they can sound alarming when heard without context. Yet many of these changes reflect adaptation rather than sudden failure.

Degenerative disc changes describe the natural changes that happen in spinal discs as we age. Over time, the discs lose some water content, become less flexible, and may show small structural changes. This process is common and does not always cause pain.

A bulging disc occurs when the outer portion of the disc extends slightly beyond its usual boundary. This does not necessarily mean the disc has ruptured. Many bulges exist without symptoms, but if nearby nerves become irritated, discomfort may arise.

A herniated disc involves a tear in the outer fibers of the disc through which the inner material may protrude. When this material presses against sensitive structures, pain can be more noticeable. Even here, the presence of herniation does not automatically determine the intensity of symptoms.

Disc thinning refers to a decrease in the height of a spinal disc, usually due to gradual fluid loss. As the space between the vertebrae becomes smaller, nearby joints and tissues may carry more load.

Sometimes disc changes are accompanied by osteophytes, or bone spurs. These are small bony projections that develop as the body attempts to stabilize areas experiencing increased stress. They represent the body's effort to adapt, even though they may contribute to stiffness.

Annular tears are small disruptions in the outer ring of the disc. While the word tear can sound severe, many such changes heal or remain symptom-free depending on how the spine is supported.

Seeing these findings together reveals an important pattern. The spine is not simply wearing out. It is responding to the demands placed upon it. These responses are part of the body's attempt to maintain stability.

Healing, therefore, does not come from protecting discs from movement, but from restoring intelligent movement to the spine. When mobility returns, effort is shared more evenly, and the surrounding muscles and joints begin to support one another effectively. Discs are then allowed to function as they were designed to.

Discs are not delicate objects waiting to fail. They are adaptable tissues that respond to how we move, rest, and live. When this is understood, fear reduces, confidence increases, and movement becomes part of recovery rather than something to be avoided.

# THE NECK AND BACK AS ONE FUNCTIONAL UNIT

Neck pain and back pain are often treated as separate problems. People speak of them as though they belong to different regions with different causes and solutions. The neck is addressed on its own, the lower back on its own, and the relationship between them is rarely considered. Yet this separation does not reflect how the body actually functions.

The spine is one continuous structure. From the base of the skull to the pelvis, it operates as a single functional unit. Movement in one region influences movement everywhere else. When one part adapts, compensates, or becomes restricted, other parts respond.

The neck does not rest on the body like an independent column. It balances on the spine, and the way the head is carried influences the curves below it. Likewise, the organization of the pelvis and lower back shapes how the head is supported above. When this relationship is harmonious, posture feels effortless. When it is disturbed, strain appears in places that may seem unrelated.

The head itself is relatively heavy and requires precise coordination to remain balanced. When it is aligned over the spine, muscular effort is minimal. But when the head drifts forward or tilts habitually, the load on the muscles increases. The neck muscles tighten to prevent collapse, and this tension often travels downward through the spine.

This is one reason neck pain frequently appears alongside upper back stiffness, shoulder discomfort, or even lower back pain. The body does not compartmentalize strain. It distributes it.

The same is true in the opposite direction. Disturbances in the pelvis or lower back often express themselves higher up. When the base becomes unstable, the spine reorganizes to maintain balance. Over time, the neck may become overworked, not because it is injured, but because it is compensating for imbalance elsewhere.

Movement patterns reinforce this unity. Whether we walk, turn, sit, or stand, the entire spine participates. If the lower spine is stiff or guarded, the neck often moves more to maintain orientation and balance. Gradually, this added demand leads to fatigue.

Breathing forms another quiet link. When breathing is shallow or restricted, the ribs move less and the neck muscles begin assisting respiration. What starts as adaptation can become chronic tension, often mistaken for a purely local neck problem.

Posture further shapes this relationship. Prolonged sitting, screen use, and habitual slouching alter the alignment between head, chest, and pelvis. Positions first adopted temporarily can slowly become the body's resting state.

Seeing the neck and back as one functional unit changes how we approach pain. Instead of asking why a single region hurts, we begin to observe how the whole spine is being used. Rather than correcting isolated segments, we look for balance across the system.

This perspective also reduces fear. When pain is viewed as a local failure, movement feels risky. When it is understood as a system-wide adaptation, movement becomes part of recovery.

Healing rarely comes from fixing one segment. It emerges as coordination is restored. When the spine begins to function as a unified structure again, load is shared more evenly, effort decreases, and pain often softens without force.

The neck and back are not separate entities. They are expressions of the same system responding to gravity, movement, and the demands of daily life. When this unity is understood, our approach to pain becomes simpler, more intelligent, and far more effective.

# THE ROLE OF MUSCLES, LIGAMENTS AND TENDONS IN SPINAL STABILITY AND PAIN

When pain arises in the back or neck, attention often turns immediately to bones, discs, or joints. Yet it is the soft tissues surrounding the spine that provide much of its day-to-day support and protection. Without understanding their role, pain can feel confusing.

Muscles are commonly thought of as structures that create movement. While this is true, their more prominent role is stabilization. Even when we are standing or sitting, muscles are quietly organizing the body against gravity. When the system is balanced, this activity is efficient and requires little effort from them. Problems begin when this activity becomes excessive or uneven.

Working alongside muscles are ligaments and tendons, two forms of connective tissue that contribute to stability in different ways. Ligaments connect bone to bone and help guide the movement of joint, while preventing excessive motion. Tendons connect muscle to bone and transmit the force generated by muscles to create movement. Together, these structures form a coordinated support network that allows the spine to remain both stable and mobile.

Muscles do not tighten randomly. They tighten in response to perceived demand. When posture is unstable, joints are restricted, or the body senses uncertainty, muscles increase their tone to provide protection. Ligaments and joint also contribute by providing passive stability, while tendons transmit the increased muscular effort required to maintain control. This is an intelligent response meant to prevent further strain.

Muscle tone refers to the gentle, continuous level of tension present in muscles even when they are not actively moving. This baseline activity is regulated by the nervous system and allows the body to maintain posture, stability, and readiness for movement. Healthy muscle tone is neither rigid nor slack; it provides quiet support so that movement can occur smoothly and efficiently. When tone becomes excessively high, muscles feel tight, or fatigued. When tone is too low, the body may feel unstable or unsupported. Balanced tone allows the spine to remain both steady and responsive.

However, when muscles are in high tone for long periods, protection turns into habit. Muscles that remain constantly engaged lose their ability to fully relax. They begin to feel tight or fatigued. Importantly, this tightness often reflects overwork rather than weakness.

Healthy muscles help maintain the natural curves of the spine and distribute load evenly. Ligaments help guide movement within safe ranges, and tendons transmit muscular force efficiently. When this system works in harmony, movement is smooth and coordinated.

When some muscles become underused, others begin to compensate, gradually creating imbalance. Muscles that remain overactive may tighten and shorten, while opposing muscles become less responsive and underutilized. This pattern often develops through repetitive movements, prolonged sitting, habitual postures, or reduced activity. As balance is lost, ligaments may become overstressed as they attempt to stabilize joints without adequate muscular support, and tendons may be subjected to repetitive strain as muscles work harder to maintain control.

As these imbalances develop, stress is no longer shared evenly across the spine. Pain often follows, not because the spine itself is damaged, but because it is functioning under distorted conditions.

One of the body's common responses to perceived spinal threat is muscle spasm. When the nervous system detects risk, such as disc irritation or instability, it signals surrounding muscles to tighten in order to restrict movement. Ligaments and joint structures contribute to this protective stiffness by limiting range, while tendons remain under continuous tension. This response is protective. It limits motion that could worsen injury. However, sustained guarding also reduces circulation, limits mobility, and increases discomfort. What began as protection becomes part of the pain experience itself.

The encouraging reality is that these soft tissue influences on pain are rarely permanent. Muscles are adaptable and trainable. Ligaments respond to improved movement patterns, and tendons adapt to balanced loading. When stability is restored thoughtfully, overactive muscles can relearn how to relax, underactive muscles can begin to participate again, and connective tissues can regain resilience.

Understanding this support system changes how we relate to tightness. It no longer appears as something to fight, but as a signal of protection and adaptation. When approached with sensitivity rather than force, the body often responds with release, improved coordination, and renewed stability.

# FASCIA AND THE HIDDEN WEB OF SUPPORT

Fascia plays an important role in how the body supports itself and adapts to stress. Without understanding fascia, pain can appear local and mechanical when it actually reflects patterns involving the whole body.

Fascia is a continuous connective tissue that surrounds and weaves through muscles, bones, organs, and nerves. It forms a body-wide network, linking distant regions into a single functional system. Through this network, tension in one area can influence many others.

Because fascia distributes force throughout the body, pain is rarely confined to a single point. A restriction in the hips can affect the lower back. Tightness around the rib cage can influence breathing. The body functions as an integrated whole.

This interconnectedness helps explain why local treatments often provide only temporary relief. Addressing one painful area without considering the broader pattern may reduce symptoms briefly, but the underlying tension often returns.

Fascia adapts to how the body is used over time. Habitual posture and repetitive movement gradually influence its structure. When the body is repeatedly held in guarded or asymmetrical positions, fascia may thicken and lose elasticity. Movement then begins to feel restricted, not necessarily because joints are damaged, but because the connective web has become less adaptable.

These changes occur slowly. By the time pain is noticed, the pattern may already be established.

Fascia is also closely linked with the nervous system. When the body perceives threat, fascial tone increases, contributing to a sense of stiffness. When the body perceives safety, fascia softens and movement becomes easier.

This relationship explains why forceful attempts to create release often provide only short-lived change. Fascia responds better to gradual loading, varied movement, and awareness.

When fascia functions well, effort is distributed more efficiently. The spine does not need to be held rigidly. Movement feels connected rather than segmented.

Pain often signals that this continuity has been reduced. Healing then becomes less about isolating tissues and more about restoring adaptability within this web of support. As adaptability returns, movement reorganizes naturally and effort decreases. The spine is supported not by bones alone, but by a living network. When this network is understood, pain begins to make sense.

# THE NERVOUS SYSTEM AND PAIN PERCEPTION

Pain is commonly assumed to be a direct signal of damage. While this may be true in acute injury, it does not explain most persistent back and neck pain. To understand pain more clearly, we must understand the role of the nervous system. The nervous system exists to protect. Pain is one of the ways it communicates perceived threat.

This means pain is not always a measure of damage. It is often a measure of protection. The nervous system continuously gathers information from posture, movement, breathing, and past experience from memory. When this combined information suggests risk, pain is produced to encourage caution.

In acute situations, this system serves us well. Pain prevents further harm. But when protective responses remain active long after tissues have healed, pain can persist.

In chronic pain, the body may no longer be injured, yet the nervous system may continue behaving as if danger is present. Muscle tone remains elevated and movement becomes guarded. The system stays in readiness even when no immediate threat exists.

Over time, sensitivity can increase. Movements that were once neutral begin to provoke pain. Fear leads to avoidance, avoidance leads to stiffness, and stiffness reinforces the sense of vulnerability.

Beliefs and expectations also influence this process. When imaging reports are misunderstood or alarming language is used, fear rises. Fear amplifies pain. The experience is real, but the system producing it has become more sensitive.

This helps explain why structural findings often fail to match symptoms. Some individuals with visible disc changes experience little pain, while others with minimal findings experience significant discomfort. Structure alone does not determine pain.

The nervous system also learns through repetition. When pain is repeatedly associated with certain movements, the system begins to anticipate danger. Pain may arise earlier, even before movement occurs. From this perspective, pain is not something to be silenced aggressively. It is something to be understood and addressed.

When the body regains a sense of safety through movement and breath, the nervous system begins to downshift. Muscle tone reduces, movement becomes less guarded, and pain often decreases naturally. The nervous system is not the enemy. It is intelligent and responsive. When it produces pain, it is attempting to help.

Understanding this, transforms the healing process. Pain is no longer seen only as a sign of damage, but as an information. And when this information is understood, the body can reorganize itself towards balance.

# WHY THE BODY FORGETS HOW TO RELAX?

Let's look deeper in to our nervous system in order to understand why body forgets to relax. Broadly, our nervous system can be understood in three parts.

The Central Nervous System, made up of the brain and spinal cord, functions as the body's command center. It processes information and guides responses.

The Peripheral Nervous System consists of the nerves that branch from the brain and spinal cord to the rest of the body. These nerves carry sensory information and support movement.

The Autonomic Nervous System regulates functions that occur without conscious effort, such as breathing, digestion, heartbeat, and blood flow. It works continuously in the background to preserve internal balance, a process known as homeostasis, where the body adjusts itself to remain stable despite changing conditions.

The autonomic system has two complementary divisions that constantly interact with one another.

The Sympathetic Nervous System prepares the body for action. Often called the fight or flight response, it is activated when a threat is perceived. Heart rate increases, breathing quickens, blood pressure rises, digestion slows, and energy becomes readily available. These changes allow the body to respond quickly when needed.

Imagine encountering a snake while walking. The body immediately prepares to freeze, flee, or protect itself. This response is useful in genuine danger. The challenge arises when the same system is activated repeatedly by everyday stress such as deadlines, traffic, emotional strain, or constant mental engagement. The body reacts similarly whether the threat is physical or psychological.

Balancing this activation is the role of the Parasympathetic Nervous System, often referred to as the rest and digest response. It slows the heart rate, normalizes breathing, supports digestion, and promotes relaxation. When this system engages, the body conserves energy and creates the internal conditions necessary for repair.

In a healthy system, activation is followed by release. Muscles contract and then relax. Effort is balanced by rest. The nervous system moves fluidly between excitation and relaxation. This rhythm allows the body to remain resilient and responsive.

Difficulties arise when activation does not resolve. When the sympathetic nervous system remains dominant for prolonged periods, the body does not simply stay alert. It begins to adapt to this heightened state as though it were normal. This adaptation is slow and often unnoticed, yet it forms the foundation for many chronic pain conditions.

This process is sometimes described as stabilization of arousal. The nervous system settles around a higher level of activation, and what was once a temporary response becomes the new baseline.

One important effect of sympathetic activation is an increase in muscle tone, the natural level of tension present in muscles even at rest. Muscle tone helps maintain posture and readiness for movement. Under stress, this tone rises so the body can respond quickly.

However, when muscles remain in a prolonged state of readiness, they lose the opportunity to fully relax. Constant tension creates compression within muscle fibers, reduces circulation, and limits recovery. As a protective measure, muscles may enter spasm to prevent further strain.

While protective at first, persistent spasm can lead to pain and restricted movement, commonly felt in the back and neck.

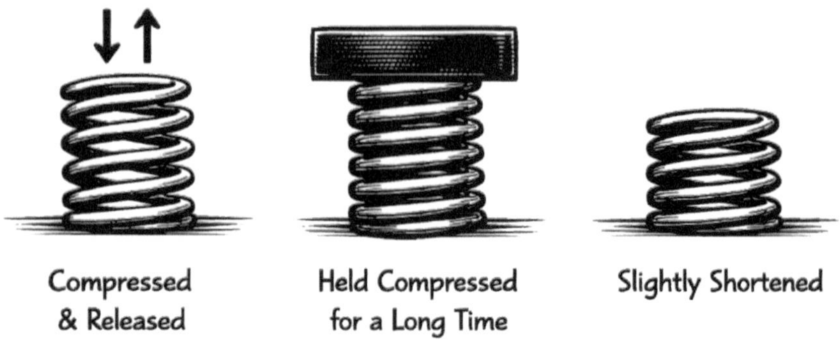


A simple example helps clarify this. Imagine a spring. When compressed and released, it returns to its original length. But if it is held compressed for a very long time, it no longer rebounds completely. It remains slightly shortened. This is not damage. It is adaptation.

The same principle applies to the human body. When the sympathetic system is repeatedly activated without sufficient recovery, muscles remain in a contracted and vigilant state. Over time, this contracted state becomes familiar. Even when a person tries to relax, the body does not fully let go. Relaxation begins to feel unfamiliar.

As this elevated tone persists, subtle shortening develops across muscles. Posture changes. Movement becomes less fluid. Joint mobility reduces. These changes often happen quietly until everyday actions begin to feel restricted.

When movement is pushed beyond this reduced range, the body responds protectively. Muscular spasms occur. Pain appears. Movements become cautious and guarded. What seems like sudden pain is usually the result of a long-standing imbalance between excitation and relaxation.

This pattern is especially visible in back and neck pain. These regions respond quickly to emotional states, breathing patterns, and postural demand. When sympathetic dominance persists, the muscles here remain continuously engaged. They do not fully soften, even during rest. Over time, the back and neck become regions of holding.

Bending, twisting, or even sustained sitting may begin to feel uncomfortable. Pain emerges not because the body is weak, but because it has been living in readiness for too long. The muscles have not forgotten how to move. They have forgotten how to rest.

If this heightened state continues, healing processes may also be affected. Since the sympathetic system suppresses functions related to repair, the body may struggle to recover fully. Circulation may become less efficient, and tissues may remain sensitive for longer.

Seen in this way, persistent tension is not simply a local muscular issue. It often reflects a nervous system that has remained in protective mode for too long. Pain, therefore, is rarely just structural. It often reflects a system that has settled into prolonged arousal.

From a yogic perspective, pain frequently represents unresolved activation rather than injury alone. It is the body's way of signaling that excitation has exceeded its capacity for release. Yoga is not always about doing more. Very often, it is about letting go of what the body has been holding unnecessarily.

Practices that encourage regulation become valuable here. Gentle breathing, mindful movement, and meditative awareness support parasympathetic activation. As the body shifts toward a calmer state, muscle tone reduces, circulation improves, and the system becomes more receptive to healing.

Healing begins not by forcing strength or flexibility, but by restoring the nervous system's ability to relax deeply. When activation and relaxation regain their natural rhythm, muscles recover their elasticity. Movement becomes freer. Effort becomes lighter. And gradually, pain begins to lose its hold.

This understanding completes the anatomical groundwork of the book. With this foundation, we can now explore how daily habits, emotional states, and conscious practices either support or interfere with the body's natural capacity to heal and adapt over time.

PART III

# HOW PAIN PATTERNS ARE CREATED

# THE POSTURAL AFTERMATH OF INJURY

When we think of injury, we usually think of pain, damage, and recovery. Once the pain reduces and imaging shows healing, we assume the chapter is over. From a yogic and biomechanical perspective, however, injury rarely ends where we think it does. The visible trauma may heal, but the body often continues to carry its consequences long after the obvious signs have disappeared.

One of the most common responses to significant injury is immobilization. Casts, braces, slings, or restricted movement are prescribed to allow bones, ligaments, or joints to heal. This immobilization is necessary and often life-saving in the short term. Yet, when a body part is not used, the muscles surrounding it weakens, joints lose mobility, and coordination declines. This is not failure. It is body intelligence responding to reduced demand.

When the cast or brace is removed, many people expect to return immediately to their previous level of function. What they often experience instead is pain. This discomfort is frequently misunderstood. The fracture may have healed and the joint may be structurally sound, yet pain persists. This is often recovery pain, discomfort arising from weakened muscles, joint stiffness, and altered movement patterns following immobilization.

The body does not label pain for us. Whether it arises from tissue injury, muscle weakness, stiffness, or compensation, it feels equally real. As a result, ongoing discomfort after injury is often mistaken as incomplete healing. This misunderstanding can lead to fear, avoidance, and further restriction of movement, deepening the problem.

A simple example illustrates this clearly. Consider someone who injures their left ankle and wears a cast for several weeks. During this time, the muscles weaken and mobility reduces. When the cast is removed, walking feels uncomfortable. To avoid pain, the person unconsciously shifts more weight onto the right leg. This feels protective and sensible. However, as weeks turn into months, the body adapts to this new pattern. The pelvis shifts, the spine adjusts, and muscles on one side begin to overwork while others underwork.

What began as a local injury slowly becomes a whole-body adaptation. If this pattern is not addressed, pain may later appear in the knee, hip, lower back, or neck. When this new pain arises, it is rarely linked to the original ankle injury. The connection has been lost in time, even though the body has been adapting continuously since the day of injury.

This is why rehabilitation is not optional. It is essential. Its purpose is not merely to reduce pain, but to restore strength, mobility, coordination, and confidence in movement. Physiotherapy and guided rehabilitation help reverse the adaptations that occurred during immobilization.

Unfortunately, rehabilitation is often rushed or discontinued once acute pain subsides. People assume normal activity will take care of the rest. The body does adapt, but it adapts to whatever patterns it is given. If compensations remain, they become reinforced and habitual.

Incomplete rehabilitation leaves the body in a state of unresolved adaptation. Muscles remain weak or tight, joints restricted, and posture altered. The individual may function reasonably well, but the system operates with imbalance. Over time, this imbalance becomes the foundation for chronic pain.

Recovery does not end when tissue heals. Healing is complete only when harmony in movement and posture is restored. Without this harmony, pain becomes a teacher rather than a symptom. Pain signals that the body has adapted in a way that no longer serves it.

Understanding the postural aftermath of injury shifts how we approach recovery. Instead of asking only whether the injury has healed, we begin to ask how the body is moving now. Is weight distributed evenly? Are certain areas overworking to protect others? Is the body still guarding against a past event?

When these questions are addressed early, recovery is smoother and more complete. When they are ignored, the injury lives on in the form of compensation and, eventually, chronic pain.

This understanding prepares us to examine the next layer of postural distortion: the subtle but powerful influence of daily habits and environments that shape the body long after injuries have been forgotten.

# LIFESTYLE, ENVIRONMENT, AND EVERYDAY POSTURAL DISTORTIONS

Not all postural distortions begin with injury. For many people, posture changes slowly and silently through daily habits that feel normal, harmless, and unavoidable. Unlike injuries, these influences do not announce themselves with pain or trauma. They shape the body gradually through repetition and routine. By the time discomfort appears, the patterns that created it are often deeply ingrained.

One of the most powerful influences on posture in modern life is a sedentary lifestyle. Many people spend a significant portion of their day sitting at desks, in cars, on sofas, or in front of screens. Sitting itself is not the problem. The difficulty arises when sitting becomes prolonged, repetitive, and poorly supported.

During long periods of sitting, especially in unsupportive chairs, slouching becomes almost inevitable. The pelvis tilts backward, the lower back loses its natural curve, and the upper back rounds forward. In this position, the spine no longer distributes gravity efficiently. Certain segments bear sustained pressure while others remain underused.

As sitting time increases, the muscles that support upright posture become less active. Guided by body intelligence, the body reduces investment in muscles that are not being used. Over time, these muscles weaken, making balanced posture more difficult. Posture deteriorates further, not because of lack of discipline, but because the body has adapted to the conditions imposed upon it.

Modern work environments intensify this pattern. Computer-based tasks often require leaning toward a screen, especially when the monitor is too low or too far away. The head shifts forward, increasing load on the neck. The shoulders round inward, and the upper back stiffens. While this posture may feel efficient briefly, maintaining it for hours places continuous strain on the cervical spine and surrounding muscles.

Neck and shoulder pain commonly arise from this pattern, yet the discomfort is rarely isolated. A forward head posture alters the balance of the entire spine. The lower back compensates, the pelvis adjusts, and muscle tension increases throughout the body. What appears to be a local problem is often a whole-body response to environmental demands.

Another overlooked factor is the loss of variety in movement. Traditional lifestyles required frequent changes in posture, including squatting, bending, walking, sitting on the floor, and standing. Contemporary environments restrict movement to a narrow range. Chairs, desks, and vehicles are designed for convenience rather than adaptability. The body, however, thrives on variation.

When movement variety is lost, some muscles remain shortened while others remain lengthened for prolonged periods. Over time, this creates imbalances in muscle tone and joint mobility. The body begins to treat these imbalanced positions as normal. When a different posture is required, discomfort may arise because the body is no longer accustomed to those movements.

Daily habits outside the workplace further reinforce these patterns. Prolonged use of mobile phones and tablets encourages bending the neck forward and rounding the shoulders. Each instance may seem minor, but repeated countless times each day, these postures reinforce strain patterns in the neck and upper back.

Multitasking adds another layer. When attention is divided, awareness of posture diminishes. People hold awkward positions longer than intended, twist while reaching, or cradle devices between shoulder and ear. Because the mind is occupied, signals of discomfort often go unnoticed.

Acute pain sometimes appears suddenly during a simple activity such as lifting, reaching, or turning. The last movement is often blamed. In reality, it merely reveals a system already overloaded by accumulated strain.

Even sitting habits influence alignment. Sitting cross-legged with one leg consistently favored shifts pelvic balance and encourages asymmetry. While occasional variation is harmless, repeated preference teaches the body to adopt uneven alignment as its default.

These everyday distortions rarely cause immediate pain. They work quietly, reshaping posture over months and years. When pain finally appears, it can feel mysterious because no single incident can be identified. The body, however, has been responding intelligently all along, adapting to the environment it inhabits.

Understanding the role of lifestyle and environment removes blame and guilt. Poor posture is not a personal failure. It is a predictable response to modern conditions. Recognizing this shifts the focus from self-criticism to intelligent change.

Healing does not require dramatic intervention. It begins with awareness. Small adjustments in how we sit, work, move, and choose supportive environments can significantly alter how the body distributes load. Introducing movement variety, reducing prolonged static postures, and restoring balance gradually reverse accumulated adaptations.

The body does not resist change. It responds to what it experiences consistently. By understanding how lifestyle and environment shape posture, we regain an active role in our physical well-being. This prepares us to explore the next dimension of postural distortion: how habitual asymmetry and unconscious choices further reinforce imbalance within the body.

# HABITUAL ASYMMETRY AND UNCONSCIOUS CHOICES

The human body is designed for balance, yet it adapts to repetition. Many postural distortions do not arise from injury or environment alone. They develop through small, repeated choices that feel comfortable, efficient, or protective. These choices are rarely deliberate. Most occur without awareness. Over time, they quietly reshape the body.

One of the most common expressions of this process is habitual asymmetry. Most people have a preferred side. They lean more on one leg while standing, carry weight on one hip, reach more often with one hand, or turn more easily in one direction. Such preferences are not inherently problematic. The body can handle asymmetry in the short term. Difficulty arises when preference becomes habit and habit becomes default.

When one side is used more consistently, the body adapts. Muscles on that side may become tighter and more dominant, while the opposite side becomes less responsive. Joints begin to experience uneven loading, the pelvis may shift subtly, and the spine adjusts to maintain balance. These changes occur gradually and often go unnoticed.

Everyday habits reinforce these patterns. Carrying a bag on the same shoulder, holding a child on the same hip, or repeatedly performing tasks on one side trains the body to distribute effort unevenly. The body adapts intelligently to repeated demand. It prioritizes efficiency, not symmetry.

An interesting consequence of long-standing asymmetry is that correction can feel uncomfortable. When someone who has lived with imbalance for years attempts to stand evenly, it may feel awkward or unnatural. This sensation is not a sign that symmetry is wrong. It simply reflects unfamiliar input. The body resists sudden change more than it resists balance.

Subtle discomfort signals are often ignored in daily life. Instead of adjusting posture or movement, we compensate quietly. Over time, these compensations accumulate. When pain eventually appears, it may seem sudden, even though the underlying patterns develop slowly.

Understanding habitual asymmetry shifts how we approach change. The goal is not to force symmetry or correct posture aggressively. Force increases tension and reinforces protection. Change begins with awareness.

Observation reveals patterns: which side we favor, how we distribute weight, and how we respond to strain. Small variations introduced consistently allow the body to reorganize gradually. The nervous system updates what feels familiar, and new patterns become easier.

Symmetry, in this context, is not rigid alignment. It is dynamic balance. The body does not require perfection. It requires options. When movement can occur in multiple directions without strain, balance has been restored.

By bringing unconscious habits into awareness, we restore those options. The body learns new patterns not through correction, but through experience.

This understanding prepares us to examine another influence on posture, the broader social and physical conditions that shape how we carry ourselves over a lifetime.

# SOCIETY, EXCESS WEIGHT AND THE SHAPING OF THE HUMAN BODY

Posture is often discussed as if it were purely mechanical, an issue of muscles, joints, and alignment. In reality, the human body develops within a social environment long before it is shaped by conscious exercise or therapy. From early childhood through adulthood, posture is influenced by expectations, routines, roles, and repeated behaviors demanded by the world around us. To understand posture fully, we must look beyond anatomy and consider the conditions in which the body is required to function.

The shaping of posture begins early in life. Young children move freely and instinctively. They squat, crawl, roll, twist, and explore using the whole body. Their movement is naturally varied, responsive, and symmetrical. They are born ambidextrous. At this stage, posture is not fixed. It changes constantly in response to social factors.

As children grow, social guidance begins to narrow this freedom. Parents and caregivers teach children how to sit, write, eat, and behave. These instructions are given with care and good intention, but they often prioritize order and conformity over natural variation. Encouraging consistent use of one hand for writing or daily tasks gradually establishes dominance patterns. Certain muscles are used repeatedly, while others receive less stimulation. Over time, this asymmetry becomes embedded in posture.

Educational environments reinforce these adaptations further. Classrooms require prolonged sitting, often in furniture that does not accommodate individual body proportions or natural spinal curves.

Children are expected to sit still, face forward, and suppress movement for long periods. While this supports learning and discipline, it limits the body's need for regular change. Muscles adapt to stillness. Joints move through fewer ranges. The spine becomes accustomed to holding rather than responding.

By adulthood, posture is no longer a moment-to-moment response. It has become a pattern.

Professional environments introduce another layer of shaping. In many workplaces, posture becomes a form of communication. Certain ways of standing, sitting, or holding the body are unconsciously associated with confidence, authority, or competence. Individuals often imitate the postures of those they admire or aspire to resemble. These adaptations may serve social or professional goals, but they are not always supportive of physical balance.

Social roles also leave a clear imprint on the body. Caregiving roles involve repeated lifting, holding, bending, and reaching. Many people habitually carry children on one side, work with the arms forward for extended periods, or spend long hours performing repetitive tasks. These movements are not inherently harmful, but when repeated without variation or recovery, they shape posture gradually and predictably.

Technology has intensified these patterns. Prolonged screen use, mobile devices, and seated work encourage forward head posture, rounded shoulders, and reduced spinal movement. The body adapts to what it does most often. Over time, these positions feel normal, even when they create strain.

Excess body weight introduces yet another layer of adaptation. Weight gain, particularly around the abdomen, shifts the center of gravity forward. To remain upright, the body compensates by leaning backward, increasing load on the lower back. Muscles redistribute effort. Spinal curves alter subtly. These changes occur gradually, often without conscious awareness.

What is important to recognize is that none of these adaptations are accidental or careless. They are intelligent responses to the demands placed on the body. Posture reflects how a person has lived, worked, learned, and adapted within their environment.

For many individuals experiencing chronic back or neck pain, these long-term adaptations explain why discomfort exists even in the absence of clear injury or structural damage. Pain emerges not from a single event, but from years of accumulated patterns that the body has learned to maintain.

Understanding the social shaping of posture prepares us to work with the body intelligently. It reminds us that healing does not require undoing life, but learning how to meet it differently.

# WHEN EMOTIONS BECOME POSTURE

Emotions are not events that occur only in the mind; they are whole-body experiences shaped by continuous interactions between neural, physiological, and behavioural processes. Modern pain science recognizes that bodily states are inseparable from emotional processing, and that perception itself is influenced by cognitive and affective factors(8)(9). Every emotion carries a physical signature that can influence muscle tone, breathing patterns, posture, and movement. Long before we consciously name what we are feeling, the body has already begun to respond(12).

This becomes evident the moment we observe posture. A slumped body with a collapsed chest and lowered head is almost universally interpreted as a sign of stress, sadness, or emotional burden. Without needing explanation, we sense that something is wrong. The body communicates emotion more honestly than words ever can.

If we encounter someone sitting in this manner, we feel an instinctive pull to check on them. Yet, if the same person were sitting upright with an open chest and relaxed spine and claimed to be deeply depressed, we would likely doubt their words. This upright posture with an open chest, we associate confidence and ease. We trust posture because it reflects the internal state directly.

Posture, therefore, is not just a mechanical arrangement of bones and muscles. It is an expression of lived experience.

When stress, anxiety, grief, or emotional strain are temporary, the body adapts and then returns to balance. The posture associated with these emotions' dissolves naturally. However, when emotional states persist, the posture that accompanies them also persists. What was once a response becomes a habit. Over time, this habit forms a structure.

This is how emotional experience slowly crystallizes into physical form.

This relationship between posture and emotion works in both directions. Emotional states influence how we hold the body. Posture, in turn, influences emotional state. A chronically collapsed posture can deepen feelings of fatigue, low mood, or lack of confidence. Restricted breathing affects nervous system regulation, making emotional resilience more difficult. This creates a feedback loop in which emotional stress shapes posture and posture reinforces emotional stress.

To understand this more deeply, we must look at how the body processes emotions in the first place.

Emotions are responses to perceived safety or threat. When an emotion arises, the nervous system immediately adjusts muscle tone, breathing, and internal readiness. The body prepares either to engage, withdraw, protect, or endure. This response happens faster than conscious thought.

Ideally, once the emotional experience passes, the nervous system returns to a baseline state. Muscles soften, breathing normalizes, and the body releases the pattern it adopted. However, when emotions are repeatedly triggered without resolution, the body does not complete this cycle.

Instead of processing emotion through expression and release, the body begins to contain it. Containment creates holding. Muscles remain partially contracted. Breathing remains shallow. The spine loses its natural buoyancy. This holding is not intentional. It is the body's attempt to stay functional while carrying emotional load.

Over time, the body learns this holding pattern as a survival strategy. The nervous system no longer distinguishes between past emotional threat and present safety. As a result, posture becomes guarded even when there is no immediate reason for protection.

This explains why emotional pain often outlives the situation that caused it. The event may be over, but the body is still holding its memory.

When emotional holding persists, it places continuous strain on the musculoskeletal system. Muscles that are not allowed to relax will eventually lose their elasticity. Joints move within reduced ranges. Movement becomes effortful rather than fluid.

Eventually, pain appears and in most cases as back or neck pain.

Their pain is real, yet medical imaging such as MRI scans may show no significant structural abnormality. This can be confusing and frustrating. However, pain does not arise only from visible damage. It often emerges from long-standing functional patterns influenced by emotion, stress, and adaptation.

From a yogic perspective, this is not an anomaly. Pain is the final expression of a body that has been holding emotional experience without release. It is the body's way of asking for attention, not at the level of structure, but at the level of experience.

In such cases, correcting posture mechanically or strengthening muscles alone offers limited relief. Without addressing the underlying emotional patterns, the body returns to its familiar holding. True change requires the body to feel safe enough to release what it has been containing(4).

When awareness is brought to posture, breath, and sensation without judgment, the body begins to soften. This is not an emotional cleansing in the dramatic sense. It is a gradual unwinding. The body learns that it no longer needs to protect itself in the same way.

As emotional holding dissolves, posture reorganizes naturally. The chest lifts without effort. The spine lengthens without force. Breathing deepens on its own. Pain often reduces, not because it was attacked, but because its purpose has been fulfilled.

Seen in this way, posture is not something to be corrected. It is something to be understood. Emotions leave their imprint on the body, but the body also holds the capacity to release them.

Pain, then, becomes not a failure of the system, but a message. When that message is listened to with patience and clarity, the body gradually finds its way back to balance.

# THE ILLUSION OF COMFORT

Modern living has dramatically changed how we relate to rest. Mattresses have become softer, pillows fluffier, and seating more cushioned than ever before. Comfort is often equated with softness. Many people believe that when they lie down, their body should sink deeply into the mattress, as though being absorbed by it. This idea feels intuitive, but it misunderstands what the human body actually needs in order to rest and heal.

The body does not relax simply because it collapses. It relaxes when it feels supported and stable. Research suggests that sleep surfaces promoting adequate support and neutral spinal alignment are associated with reduced back pain and improved sleep quality[13][14].

At a fundamental level, the body is always seeking grounding. We can observe this while walking. When the surface beneath the feet is stable, movement feels effortless. When it is unstable, muscular effort increases as the body makes constant adjustments to maintain balance. Biomechanical research similarly emphasizes that spinal stability is essential for efficient load transfer and for preventing excessive micro-movements that may contribute to pain[15].

The same principle applies when we sit or lie down. When the body meets a surface, it instinctively looks for reliability. Stability allows muscles to release. When stability is absent, muscles remain subtly alert, making continuous micro-adjustments. This process is unconscious but significant over time.

Very soft mattresses, cushions, and seats often fail to provide grounding. Instead of supporting the body evenly, they allow it to sink asymmetrically.

The pelvis tilts. The spine adapts to the surface beneath it. Importantly, these surfaces do not create new imbalances. They amplify those already present.

Even slight asymmetries become exaggerated on overly soft surfaces. The body sinks into its dominant patterns, and over time those patterns are reinforced rather than corrected.

Clinical research supports the importance of appropriate mattress firmness. A randomized controlled trial found that individuals with chronic low back pain reported less pain and disability when sleeping on a medium-firm mattress compared to a very firm one[(14)], while systematic review evidence suggests that mattresses balancing comfort with support are most favorable for spinal health[(13)].

This is why, in acute back pain, people are sometimes advised to rest on a flat, firm surface. The intention is not discomfort but stability. A firm surface supports the body evenly, allowing muscles to release fully.

When the surface is too soft, the opposite occurs. Muscles remain subtly active, adjusting to constant shifts in support. The body searches for stability that it never quite finds. What is meant to be rest becomes another form of work.

This low-grade muscular activity prevents full recovery. Instead of allowing the nervous system to downshift, it maintains a background level of alertness that contributes to fatigue, stiffness, and pain.

True comfort, therefore, is not softness alone. It is the combination of support and stability that allows the body to feel safe enough to let go.

The effects of excessive softness become more evident in daily habits. Beds have become reading spaces, workstations, and lounging areas. Sofas and cushions are used for hours without attention to alignment.

Consider sitting on a bed while reading or working on a laptop. The pelvis sinks backward, the spine rounds, and the head moves forward. Although this posture feels comfortable initially, it places continuous strain on the back and neck. The problem is not a single instance but repetition.

When repeated daily, the body begins to accept this position as normal. Muscles adapt accordingly[15], and the spine reorganizes around the habit.

Soft seating has similar effects. When sitting on highly cushioned chairs or sofas, the body often sinks unevenly. People lean to one side or slouch without noticing. Because the surface gives way, the body lacks a clear reference for alignment and compensates continuously.

Pillows also influence alignment. Very soft or excessively thick pillows can distort the position of the neck during sleep. When the head is pushed forward or allowed to sink unevenly, the cervical spine remains misaligned for hours. Night after night, this contributes to neck stiffness, headaches, and upper back discomfort.

The body does not distinguish between daytime and nighttime strain. Prolonged distortion during sleep accumulates just as postural stress does during waking hours.

What makes these habits challenging is their invisibility. People believe they are resting and being kind to their bodies. In reality, the body is continually stabilizing and adjusting.

Awareness therefore becomes essential. Cushions, pillows, and beds are not inherently harmful. The issue lies in excess softness, prolonged use, and lack of attention to posture. A surface should support the body rather than amplify imbalances. It should provide enough firmness for grounding while offering comfort without collapse.

When the body finds stable support, muscles release naturally. Breathing deepens and the nervous system settles. Eventually, healing becomes possible.

Comfort must be redefined. It is not the feeling of sinking away, but the presence of support that allows the body to rest in natural alignment.

Healing does not always begin with complex interventions. Sometimes it begins with questioning everyday choices. Where we sit, how we lie down, and what we rest upon influence the body far more than we often realize.

# FOOTWEAR AND IT'S RELATION TO BACK OR NECK PAIN

The feet are the body's first point of contact with the ground. Every step we take sends information upward through the legs, pelvis, and spine, shaping posture, balance, and movement. Specialized receptors in the feet contribute to proprioception by signalling body position and movement to the nervous system[16]. Yet, when back pain or neck pain is discussed, the feet are rarely considered. Attention is directed toward the spine, the discs, or the muscles of the back, while the foundation on which the entire system rests is largely ignored.

This oversight is significant.

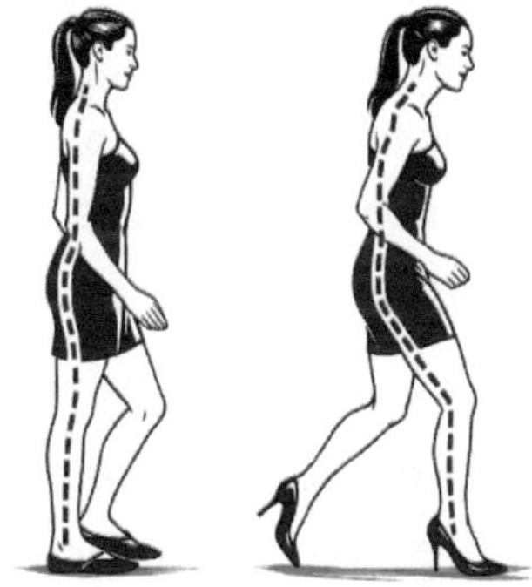

High heels elevate the heels above the forefoot, forcing the feet into an unnatural position. This shifts body weight forward toward the toes and alters the body's center of gravity. To prevent falling forward, the body compensates. The pelvis tilts, and the lower back often arches more than normal. This exaggerated arch in the lower back increases compressive load on the lumbar spine and places additional strain on the muscles supporting it.

These changes do not remain limited to the lower back. As pelvic alignment shifts, the entire spine adapts. Abdominal muscles lose effective engagement, while lower back muscles shorten and tighten. Over time, this imbalance alters how forces are distributed through the body, increasing the risk of chronic discomfort.

Walking in high heels requires continuous muscular effort to maintain balance. The calves remain in a shortened position, ankle mobility reduces, and the natural shock absorption of the feet is compromised. With repeated use, the body adapts to these conditions. Even when high heels are not worn, residual tension and altered posture may persist.

Occasional use may not cause lasting harm. However, regular use over long periods teaches the body to manage gravity inefficiently. The body does not resist these changes. It adapts to them, treating the altered alignment as normal. This is why long-term use of high heels is often associated with lower back pain, hip discomfort, and knee issues. Many women who approach therapy complain about these issues and yet ignorantly use high heels.

Modern footwear, particularly heavily cushioned shoes, alters how the body interacts with the ground. Thick soles, and soft cushioning, are designed to absorb impact and increase comfort. While this may reduce immediate sensation under the feet, it also reduces the amount of information reaching the nervous system. The foot contains a dense network of sensory receptors that detect pressure, texture, and load. Research demonstrates that these sensory input plays an important role in balance and coordinated movement[(16)].

When footwear dampens this feedback, the nervous system receives a less accurate picture of the ground. The body may still move, but it moves with reduced clarity. Subtle adjustments that normally occur automatically become delayed or exaggerated. Stability is achieved not through fine coordination, but through increased muscular effort higher up the chain.

This is why people often feel more "supported" in cushioned shoes, yet paradoxically develop greater postural instability over time. Studies comparing habitually barefoot and shoe runners show that footwear alters foot strike patterns and collision forces, thereby changing how loads travel through the body[(17)].

Reduced sensory input from the feet shifts the burden of balance upward. The ankles stiffen. The knees lock. The hips lose fluidity. The pelvis begins to tilt or rotate to compensate. The spine, sitting atop this altered foundation, responds by increasing tension in certain regions to maintain upright posture. What begins as a change at the level of the feet slowly expresses itself as discomfort in the lower back, mid-back, or neck.

Barefoot awareness offers a contrasting experience. When the foot makes direct contact with the ground, sensory feedback increases dramatically. Pressure changes, weight shifts, and subtle movements are immediately detected. The nervous system responds by refining coordination rather than increasing effort. Muscles engage only as much as needed. Posture becomes more responsive and less rigid. Emerging research also suggests that reduced footwear can strengthen intrinsic foot muscles, potentially improving foot function[(18)].

This does not mean that everyone should abandon footwear entirely. Rather, it highlights the importance of sensory awareness. Even brief periods of barefoot standing or walking, when done safely, can help reawaken the foot's role in postural regulation. Yoga practices that emphasize grounding through the feet cultivate this awareness deliberately. Standing asanas, when approached with attention to foot contact and weight distribution, reconnect the entire postural chain.

The connection between the feet, pelvis, and spine is therefore not purely mechanical but functional. The foot informs the pelvis how to organize itself. The pelvis determines how the spine stacks and moves. When the feet are disconnected from the ground, the pelvis often loses its sense of orientation. This can lead to excessive anterior or posterior tilt, asymmetrical loading, or habitual gripping in the hip muscles. The spine adapts accordingly, often developing patterns of tension that are later interpreted as back or neck pain.

From a yogic perspective, grounding is not merely symbolic but physiological. Clear sensory input allows the body to distribute load more efficiently, reducing the need for unnecessary muscular bracing.

Footwear that prioritizes softness and insulation over sensory feedback may feel comfortable in the short term, but over time it can contribute to diminished postural intelligence. This does not imply that cushioned shoes are inherently harmful. It suggests that constant reliance on them, without counterbalancing practices that restore foot awareness, can subtly influence posture and movement in ways that affect the spine.

Back or neck pain often reflects a loss of communication within the system rather than a failure of structure. Reestablishing the dialogue between the feet and the ground is one way of restoring that communication. When the feet remember how to sense, the pelvis learns how to balance. When the pelvis balances, the spine no longer needs to strain.

Sometimes, the path to easing back or neck pain begins not with focusing exclusively on the spine, but with paying closer attention to the ground beneath our feet.

# MOBILE PHONES, SCREENS, AND NECK PAIN

Neck pain has become one of the most common physical complaints of modern life, and mobile phones and screens are often blamed as the primary culprits[19]. The term "text neck" is now widely used to describe the forward bending of the neck while looking down at a phone. While neck angle does matter, focusing only on posture oversimplifies the problem and misses the deeper mechanisms through which screen use affects the body.

Neck pain associated with screen use is not merely a mechanical issue. Contemporary clinical understanding recognizes that neck pain is influenced by an interplay of biomechanical, psychological, and behavioral factors rather than posture alone[6].

When we look at a screen, especially a small handheld one, our attention narrows. The eyes fixate, the breath subtly changes, and the nervous system shifts into a state of sustained focus. This state is not inherently harmful. The problem arises when it is held for long periods without interruption. The body begins to organize itself around this attentional demand.

As attention becomes sustained, breathing often becomes less variable, and muscles of the neck and shoulders may increase their activity to stabilize the head and support visual focus. Experimental research has demonstrated that demanding visual tasks can elevate trapezius muscle activation, even in otherwise low-load physical environments[20]. This increased tone is typically reflexive rather than conscious.

Eye strain plays a significant role in this process. The muscles that control eye movement and focus are neurologically linked to the muscles of the neck. Prolonged visual effort, especially on close-range screens, increases demand on this system. As the eyes tire, the neck muscles work harder to stabilize the head and maintain visual clarity. Over time, this creates a pattern of chronic tension that persists even when the screen is no longer present.

The posture associated with screen use is often described as forward head posture. Mechanical studies show that as the head moves anteriorly, the load experienced by the cervical spine increases substantially(9). However, this posture is not merely the result of poor alignment. It is the body's attempt to bring the eyes closer to the object of attention. The head moves forward not because the neck is weak, but because the nervous system prioritizes visual engagement over postural efficiency.

This helps explain why correcting neck position alone often provides incomplete relief. Even with improved alignment, discomfort may persist if sustained attention, limited movement variability, and ongoing muscular activation remain unaddressed(6).

Screen use also alters nervous system tone. Prolonged interaction with digital devices tends to increase sympathetic nervous system activity. This manifests as heightened alertness, subtle stress, and increased muscle tone, particularly in the neck, shoulders, and jaw(21). Over time, the system loses its ability to return easily to a relaxed state. Muscles that were meant to respond briefly remain partially contracted even at rest.

This sustained tone affects the cervical spine significantly. The neck, designed for mobility and responsiveness, becomes stiff and guarded. Small movements feel effortful. Turning the head may produce discomfort or a sense of resistance. Pain emerges not because the neck is damaged, but because it has been held in a state of prolonged readiness.

From a yogic perspective, attention is not just neutral. Where attention goes, prana follows. When attention is consistently drawn outward into screens, the body organizes itself accordingly. Breath becomes secondary and sensory awareness narrows. Over time, these disconnect between awareness and the body contributes to pain.

Restoring balance requires more than ergonomic adjustments. While screen height and posture matter, they are insufficient on their own. What is needed is periodic release of visual focus, conscious restoration of breath, and deliberate reorientation of attention back into the body. Even brief moments of lifting the gaze, softening the eyes, and allowing the breath to deepen can interrupt the cycle of tension.

Yoga addresses these mechanisms directly. Practices that coordinate breath with movement recalibrate nervous system tone. Gentle neck movements restore mobility without force. Practices that emphasize visual relaxation, such as closing the eyes or soft gaze, or yogic practices such as Trataka reduce the load on the cervical system. Over time, the neck relearns that it does not need to hold itself rigid to remain safe.

Neck pain associated with screens is not a failure of discipline or posture. It is the body's intelligent response to sustained attentional demand in an environment that rarely invites pause. When we understand this, the solution shifts from correction to awareness.

Reducing neck pain in the digital age is not about avoiding screens altogether. It is about learning how to use them without losing the body in the process. When attention, breath, and posture are brought back into conversation, the neck no longer needs to carry the burden alone.

# SKELETAL IRREGULARITIES AND THE MYTH OF FIXITY

When people speak about back pain or neck pain or spinal discomfort, they often refer to skeletal irregularities. Terms such as lordosis, kyphosis, flat back, or scoliosis are commonly used, sometimes casually and sometimes with concern. These terms describe variations in the natural curves of the spine, and while they may sound alarming, they are far more common than most people realize.

As we have read earlier, human spine is not meant to be straight. From the side, it naturally forms a gentle double S-shaped curve that allows the body to distribute load efficiently, absorb shock, and adapt to movement[(22),(15)]. When this natural curvature changes beyond a certain range, it is described as a skeletal irregularity. In some individuals, the lower back curve becomes exaggerated. In others, the upper back rounds excessively. Some people lose the natural curves almost entirely, resulting in a flat back. There are also cases where the spine appears straight when viewed from the side but shows a lateral deviation when seen from the back. Even when the spine looks straight externally, it may still be structurally distorted.

These variations are widespread. Some are present from birth, reflecting the natural uniqueness of each individual. No two spines are identical, and the degree of curvature we develop depends on genetics, growth patterns, and how we adapt to gravity as we grow into adulthood[(15)]. At the same time, an increasing number of people develop these changes later in life. These are not congenital conditions. They emerge gradually, often without the person being aware of the change until discomfort or pain begins to appear.

To understand why this happens, it is important to look beyond bones. Bones do not move on their own. They respond to forces applied to them. Along the spine, muscles create continuous patterns of pull. When these patterns are balanced, the spine maintains its natural alignment. When they are not, the spine adapts accordingly(22).

Prolonged postural habits, asymmetrical movement patterns, emotional holding, and sustained muscular tension all create uneven forces along the spinal column. Over time, these forces begin to reshape posture. The spine does not resist this process. It adapts to the demands placed upon it. This adaptation happens slowly and quietly, often over years. Eventually, what was once a temporary posture becomes a structural tendency(23)(22).

This understanding, challenges a common belief that spinal structures cannot be changed. Many people are told that once the spine develops an irregular curve, it is permanent and must simply be managed. This belief often leads to fear, resignation, and overdependence on external interventions.

While it is true that the skeletal system changes more slowly than muscles, rigidity does not mean immutability. Bones are living tissues. They respond to long-term mechanical forces, loading patterns, and changes in muscular tension(23). If irregular muscular pull can gradually move the spine away from its optimal alignment, it is reasonable to question why balanced muscular engagement cannot guide it back toward a healthier structure.

Structural change in the skeleton does not happen quickly. It requires patience, consistency, and intelligent practice. The goal is not to force the spine into a particular shape, but to remove the forces that are constantly distorting it. When muscles begin to function more evenly, the spine is no longer pulled in conflicting directions. Over time, this allows the skeletal system to adapt towards balance.

Many individuals have experienced meaningful improvements in spinal alignment through sustained and mindful work. These changes are not dramatic or sudden, but they are real. The skeleton responds last, but it does respond.

Viewing the body through this lens fundamentally changes how structural variations are interpreted. Skeletal irregularities are no longer seen as fixed defects, but as expressions of adaptation. And what has adapted once can adapt again. When approached with understanding rather than force, the body reveals a remarkable capacity for reorganization and healing.

If the skeleton is capable of adapting and even changing over time, a natural question arises. What is it responding to every single day?

The answer lies not in dramatic events, but in repetition.

Skeletal irregularities do not appear suddenly. They are rarely the result of a single posture or isolated incident. In most cases, they are the outcome of patterns that are repeated so often that the body begins to treat them as normal. What the body does repeatedly, it learns. What it learns, it begins to embody.

Every posture we take, whether sitting, standing, walking, or lying down, places a specific demand on the body. When that posture is temporary, the body adapts and then returns to balance. But when the same posture is repeated daily, for hours at a time, the body begins to organize itself around it.

This is how occasional posture may contribute to long-term structural adaptation.

Most people do not hold one harmful posture continuously. Instead, they repeat small, seemingly insignificant patterns. Sitting with a slight slouch. Leaning consistently to one side. Standing with weight shifted habitually onto one leg. Holding the head forward while looking at screens. None of these appear alarming on their own. Yet the body does not measure impact in moments. It measures it in duration and frequency.

Muscles adapt first. They learn which positions are expected of them and begin to maintain those positions with minimal effort. Over time due to body intelligence, muscles that are repeatedly shortened remain shortened, while those that are rarely engaged lose responsiveness. This creates imbalance, not because the body is failing, but because it is adapting efficiently to the demands placed upon it[15].

Once muscular imbalance stabilizes, the skeleton begins to follow. Bones respond to long-term mechanical forces. Joints remodel themselves to support habitual ranges of movement. The spine adjusts its curves to sustain what has become the dominant pattern[23].

At this stage, posture no longer feels like something we are doing. It feels like who we are.

This is why simply instructing someone to sit or stand correctly rarely leads to lasting change. The body cannot hold a posture that it has not learned to inhabit. Without addressing the patterns that shaped the posture, any correction feels forced and collapses as soon as attention shifts.

Pain often emerges at this point. Not because the body is broken, but because it has adapted too narrowly. When movement is required outside familiar patterns, strain arises. The body resists not movement itself, but unfamiliar movement.

Understanding this, reframes the entire approach to healing. The question shifts from how to correct a posture to how posture was learned. The body must be offered new experiences before it can adopt new structures.

This also explains why meaningful change takes time. Structural adaptation is cautious by nature. The body does not reorganize itself in response to intention alone. It reorganizes itself in response to consistent and repeated input.

Seen in this light, skeletal irregularities are not fixed problems. They are records of repetition written into the body. When repetition changes, structure begins to change as well.

# DISC BULGE DOES NOT AUTOMATICALLY MEAN PAIN

One of the most common and deeply ingrained beliefs around back or neck pain is the idea that a disc bulge automatically equals pain. For many people, the moment they read the words *disc bulge*, *disc protrusion*, or *disc degeneration* on an MRI report, pain suddenly acquires a clear and frightening explanation. The scan appears to offer certainty. Something is visible; therefore, something must be wrong.

The reality is far more subtle.

As we discussed in the earlier chapters of the book, large scientific studies have consistently shown that disc bulges and other structural changes in the spine are extremely common in people who have no back pain at all. One of the earliest and most influential studies by Jensen and colleagues examined MRI scans of adults with no history of back pain and found that a significant percentage had disc bulges, disc degeneration, and even herniations despite being completely symptom-free[(24)]. Later, a large systematic review by Brinjikji and colleagues confirmed these findings across multiple age groups, showing that imaging features commonly labeled as "degenerative" are often part of normal human aging rather than indicators of disease or damage[(1)].

If disc bulges were sufficient by themselves to cause pain, a majority of adults would be suffering constantly. Yet many individuals with clear disc changes live active, functional, and pain-free lives. This alone tells us something essential: structural change and pain are not the same thing.

Pain is not generated by discs in isolation. Pain is an experience produced by the nervous system, shaped by how the body moves, how muscles coordinate, how posture is maintained, how stress is processed, and how safe or threatened the system feels. As Bogduk explains in his detailed review on the physiology of back pain, pain can arise from multiple mechanisms and does not map reliably to structural findings seen on imaging[25].

MRI reports, however, can unintentionally amplify pain by altering perception. Medical terminology, though precise, is often interpreted emotionally. Words such as bulge, tear, or degeneration suggest fragility and damage to the untrained reader. This creates fear when not explained properly. Fear changes movement. People begin to guard, stiffen, avoid certain positions, and reduce activity. Muscles tighten, coordination declines, and the nervous system becomes more vigilant.

Ironically, it is often this protective response, rather than the disc itself, that intensifies pain.

Research has shown that imaging findings, frequently leads to overdiagnosis and overtreatment, particularly when structural changes are assumed to be the primary cause of pain without considering functional and psychosocial factors[26]. Clinical guidelines now caution against relying on imaging alone to guide treatment decisions, especially in the absence of serious neurological signs[27].

Modern pain science further clarifies this distinction. Pain is not a direct measure of tissue damage. It is a protective output of the nervous system, influenced by perceived threat, past experience, beliefs, and context. Moseley and others have shown that pain can persist long after tissues have healed, or even appear in the absence of ongoing injury, due to heightened sensitivity within the nervous system[28]. Practical guidelines for explaining chronic musculoskeletal pain emphasize that central sensitization and learned protective responses can maintain pain without ongoing structural pathology[29].

This understanding changes how we interpret disc findings. A disc bulge may exist quietly for years without symptoms. Pain often emerges when the surrounding system becomes sensitized, overloaded, or fearful. The disc itself may not change at all, yet the experience of pain can increase dramatically.

From a yogic perspective, the body is not a static structure waiting to fail. It is a living, adaptive system. Discs respond to load, movement, and hydration. Muscles reorganize based on use. The nervous system continuously recalibrates based on experience and perceived safety. When movement is restored gradually and confidence returns, pain often reduces even though the disc bulge remains unchanged.

This does not deny the existence of disc-related pain. There are situations where disc pathology clearly contributes to symptoms, particularly when neurological signs such as progressive weakness or loss of sensation are present. However, extensive research comparing surgical and non-surgical approaches has shown that many people with disc herniation improve over time with conservative care, and that imaging findings alone are not sufficient to justify invasive intervention[30][31].

When we separate structure from sensation, images from lived experience, and fear from function, the path forward becomes clearer. Pain becomes something to understand rather than something to fear. Movement becomes a tool for recovery rather than a threat to avoid.

A disc bulge may be visible on a scan. Healing, however, depends on how the entire system learns to move, respond, and feel safe again.

# HOW THE BODY LEARNS ALIGNMENT THROUGH FEEDBACK

The body does not learn alignment through instruction alone. It learns through experience. Every movement, every posture, and every interaction with the environment provides feedback. Over time, this feedback teaches the body what feels stable, what feels efficient, and what feels safe[16].

Alignment is not something the body calculates intellectually. It is something the body senses. From early childhood, the nervous system learns to organize posture by responding to gravity, ground reaction, and internal sensation[16][32]. When a child stands, falls, adjusts, and stands again, the body gathers information. Muscles learn how much effort is required. Joints learn where support is available. Balance emerges not from effort, but from repeated feedback[32]. This process continues throughout life. The body constantly monitors pressure, tension, and ease. When a posture allows the body to feel supported, breathing remains free and muscles soften. When a posture creates strain or instability, muscles tighten and breathing changes. These signals are subtle, but they are continuous[32].

Over time, the body begins to prefer postures that feel predictable and manageable, even if they are not optimal.

This is where alignment begins to drift. If the feedback the body receives is distorted, alignment adapts accordingly. Sitting on unstable or overly soft surfaces, holding the body in asymmetrical positions, or repeatedly moving with poor support alters the sensory information the body relies on. The nervous system learns to stabilize around these conditions. What feels familiar becomes normal. What feels normal becomes correct, even if it is inefficient.

The body does not ask whether a posture is ideal. It asks whether it is survivable. This explains why people often feel uncomfortable when they first attempt to correct their posture. A more aligned position may feel unfamiliar, effortful, or even wrong. Not because it is harmful, but because it does not match the body's learned expectations. The nervous system interprets unfamiliarity as instability[33].

Feedback is the language through which this learning happens. When the feet receive clear pressure from the ground, the legs organize themselves naturally. When the pelvis feels evenly supported, the spine stacks itself with less effort. When the head balances effortlessly over the spine, neck muscles relax. These are not conscious corrections. They are automatic responses to accurate sensory input.

Conversely, when feedback is unclear or inconsistent, the body compensates. Muscles grip, joints lock and posture stiffens. The body chooses tension over uncertainty.

True alignment emerges when feedback changes. When the body is placed in environments and positions that provide clear, stable information, the nervous system reorganizes naturally. Muscles release where they no longer need to hold. Support redistributes itself through the skeletal system. Alignment improves not because it is forced, but because it is felt[16].

This also explains why awareness is such a powerful tool. When attention is brought to sensation without judgment, feedback becomes clearer. The body begins to recognize unnecessary tension. Small adjustments arise spontaneously. Posture shifts subtly, not through command, but through recognition.

Over time, repeated exposure to accurate feedback rewires the body's sense of normal. Alignment becomes easier to maintain because it no longer feels foreign. It feels familiar. The body has learnt it[33].

This learning process requires patience. Feedback-based change is gradual, because the nervous system values consistency over intensity. Short bursts of correction followed by long periods of habitual posture do little to alter alignment. What matters is the quality of information the body receives again and again.

When the body is given consistent experiences of stability, support, and ease, it adapts. Muscles reorganize. Movement becomes more fluid. Posture softens without collapse. Pain often reduces as the body no longer needs to protect itself through tension.

In this way, alignment is not something imposed from outside. It is something rediscovered from within.

The nervous system has the capacity to reorganize. It simply needs the right feedback to remember.

PART IV

# THE TREATMENT ILLUSION

# SURGERY AND THE QUESTION OF IRREVERSIBILITY

Before speaking about surgery, it is important to acknowledge a recurring experience that has shaped my understanding of this subject.

Many people come to me when they are standing at the threshold of a decision. They arrive carrying an MRI report, often accompanied by fear and confusion. They have been advised surgery for a spinal issue and are unsure how to proceed. Others come after surgery has already been performed, seeking relief from pain that has either returned or changed its form. In both cases, the questions they ask are strikingly similar.

They ask whether surgery was truly necessary. They ask whether something else could have been tried. They ask why pain persists even though the structure has been altered.

These individuals are not careless or uninformed. Most are responsible, thoughtful people trying to make the best decision with the information available to them. They are often pressed for time, under professional or family obligations, and genuinely seeking relief. Surgery is presented to them as a clear solution, backed by imaging and medical authority. Faced with ongoing discomfort and limited options, many feel they have little choice but to agree.

What becomes apparent, however, when listening carefully to their stories, is that the decision for surgery is rarely made in a spacious or reflective state. It is often made under pressure. Pressure from pain. Pressure from urgency. Pressure from the belief that the body is damaged and must be fixed quickly.

Those who come after surgery often describe an initial sense of relief. Pain may reduce. Mobility may return. Life appears to resume. Yet, with time, new challenges emerge. Stiffness appears in unfamiliar places. Pain shifts rather than disappears. Movement feels restricted in ways that were not anticipated. When this happens, confusion deepens, because the problem was believed to have been resolved permanently.

Those who come before surgery often sense, intuitively, that something is missing from the conversation. They may have been shown images of discs and vertebrae, but they have not been helped to understand their body as a whole. They feel that the focus has been placed entirely on structure, while their lived experience remains unexplored.

It is from listening to these stories, repeated over years, that the need for caution becomes clear. Surgery is not merely a medical procedure. It is a decision that permanently alters the relationship between structure, movement, and adaptation. Once that change is made, the body must reorganize itself around it for the rest of one's life.

What follows is not an argument against surgery, but an invitation to understand it more completely. Only when we see surgery within the broader context of how the body functions, adapts, and compensates can we make decisions that are informed rather than rushed.

Surgery has become a common recommendation for spinal issues. Disc bulges, disc degeneration, and structural changes visible on imaging often lead people to believe that surgical correction is necessary. The decision is frequently driven by what appears on an MRI rather than by the lived experience of the individual[(24)].

What is rarely discussed with enough depth is the meaning of these findings.

As discussed earlier, multiple studies have shown that a significant percentage of healthy, pain-free adults display disc bulges, disc degeneration, and other structural changes on spinal imaging. In some studies, fifty to sixty percent of asymptomatic individuals show findings that are often labeled as pathological. These individuals have no pain, no limitation, and no functional impairment, yet their scans resemble those of people who are suffering[1].

This raises an important question. If structural changes alone were sufficient to cause pain, why are so many people functioning normally despite these findings?

Understanding this, changes how we interpret imaging. The spine is not an isolated structure. It is part of a complex system involving muscles, fascia, nervous system regulation, movement patterns, and emotional holding. Pain arises from the interaction of these systems, not from structure alone[25]

When surgery is recommended based primarily on imaging, without adequate consideration of these other factors, the risk of unnecessary intervention increases[30].

This does not mean surgery is never required. There are clear situations where surgical intervention is necessary and life-changing. However, in many cases, surgery is recommended as a first or early option rather than a last resort[26].

The reason this deserves caution is simple. Surgery creates irreversible change.

When a disc is removed or fused, that segment of the spine permanently loses mobility. The body adapts, as it always does. Movement that once occurred at that segment is redistributed to adjacent segments. These segments then work harder to compensate. Over time, this increased demand can lead to further degeneration, pain, or dysfunction elsewhere in the spine[34].

The body does not forget what has been removed. Once structural mobility is lost, it cannot be reclaimed. Muscles can be trained. Movement patterns can be changed. Nervous system regulation can improve. But a surgically altered structure remains altered for life[35].

This is why the decision to undergo spinal surgery must be approached with patience and discernment. It is not merely about resolving current pain. It is about understanding how the body will function decades later.

One of the most common reasons people opt for surgery today is not the severity of their condition, but the lack of time. Working on the body through movement, rehabilitation, or therapeutic practice requires sustained effort and patience. It demands attention, consistency, and personal involvement. Surgery, by contrast, appears efficient. A procedure completed within a day, followed by rapid discharge and early mobility, creates the impression of a quick and definitive solution.

Advances in surgical techniques have shortened recovery periods. This has further increased the temptation to intervene early. If pain can be reduced in days rather than months, the choice can seem obvious, especially in a culture that values speed and productivity[(31)].

> ***What is often overlooked is that speed of recovery does not equal depth of healing.***

Early reduction in pain does not guarantee long-term stability. The absence of pain immediately after surgery does not mean that the underlying patterns contributing to the problem have been addressed. In many cases, these patterns remain unchanged. The body adapts around a new structural limitation rather than resolving the original dysfunction[(30)].

When surgery is chosen primarily because there is no time to work on oneself, the long-term cost may far exceed the short-term relief. Studies that followed patients for several years show that, in many spinal conditions, people who have surgery and those who do not often end up with similar long-term results, even though surgery usually improves symptoms faster at first[(31)].

This is why it is essential to seek multiple opinions before deciding on surgery. Consulting different medical professionals, physiotherapists, and movement-based or rehabilitative practitioners allows for a more comprehensive understanding of the condition. Exploring conservative options first is not a rejection of medicine. It is an acknowledgement of the body's capacity to adapt when given appropriate conditions and time.

Only when all reasonable non-invasive approaches have been explored, and when quality of life remains severely compromised, does surgery become a considered and informed choice rather than a reaction.

The body deserves time. Healing is not always fast, but it is often deep.

Choosing to delay a surgery when possible is not indecision. It is responsibility. It reflects respect for the complexity of the human system and for the irreversible nature of structural intervention.

In India, it is common for people to consult an orthopaedic surgeon as the very first step when they experience pain. Access to specialists is relatively easy, and seeking expert opinion is seen as responsible and efficient.

While this approach is understandable, it subtly shapes the direction of care from the very beginning.

An orthopaedic surgeon is trained to look at structure. Their expertise lies in bones, joints, discs, and surgical correction. When pain is presented to them, it is naturally interpreted through this lens. Imaging is ordered, structural findings are identified, and treatment options are discussed accordingly.

What often remains unexplored at this stage are movement patterns, muscular imbalances, breathing habits, nervous system regulation, and the cumulative effects of daily posture and lifestyle. These factors may not appear on scans, yet they play a central role in how pain develops and persists.

This does not reflect a limitation of the surgeon, but the nature of specialization itself.

When the journey begins with structure, the solution is often sought in structure. As a result, conservative approaches such as physiotherapy, therapeutic movement, Yoga therapy or other such guided practices may be considered only after pain has persisted or interventions have failed.

Reversing this sequence can be meaningful. Beginning with a physical therapist or movement-based practitioner allows the body to be assessed functionally before being labeled structurally. Many issues can be addressed at this level, sometimes reducing pain significantly and clarifying whether surgical consultation is truly necessary.

When surgery is eventually considered, it is then done from a position of clarity rather than urgency.

This is not about choosing one system over another. It is about choosing the right sequence. Structure matters. Surgery has its place. When the question asked is "How is the body functioning?" and not "what is wrong with the spine?", then the range of possibilities expand.

A thoughtful beginning often prevents a rushed ending. Surgery may sometimes be necessary but decision should be taken only after ruling out all the other options.

## Before You Decide on Surgery

Before making a decision that permanently alters the structure of the body, it is worth pausing.

Ask yourself whether your pain has been explored beyond what appears on imaging. Have posture, movement habits, breathing patterns, emotional stress, and daily routines been examined with the same seriousness as the MRI report?

Consider how long you have truly worked with conservative approaches. Have you given your body sufficient time to respond to rehabilitation, therapeutic movement, or guided practice, or has urgency driven the timeline?

Reflect on whether the recommendation for surgery arose from clear neurological compromise or from persistent discomfort that has not yet been approached holistically.

Ask how many perspectives you have heard. Have you sought opinions from more than one medical professional? Have you spoken to physiotherapists or movement-based therapists such as Yoga therapists who understand how the body adapts outside of surgical intervention?

Examine your relationship with time. Are you choosing surgery because it feels like the fastest solution, or because all reasonable alternatives have been explored and exhausted?

Ask yourself how well you understand the long-term implications. Do you know what mobility will be lost, how the body may compensate, and how this change could influence movement decades later?

Notice your emotional state while deciding. Is the decision being made from fear, pressure, or exhaustion, or from clarity and understanding?

Finally, ask whether you feel informed rather than rushed. A considered decision is not a delayed one. It is one that allows space for understanding.

Surgery may sometimes be necessary. When it is chosen, let it be chosen with awareness rather than urgency.

# CALCIUM, BONE HEALTH, AND THE QUESTION OF SUPPLEMENTATION

One of the most common recommendations people receive when concerns about bone health arise is to start calcium tablets. Calcium is widely associated with strong bones, and the idea that more calcium automatically leads to better skeletal health has become deeply ingrained. As a result, many people begin supplementation without questioning whether their body actually needs it or how it processes calcium in different forms.

Recent research, however, invites us to look at this assumption more carefully.

Several large studies comparing calcium intake from food with calcium intake from supplements have shown an important distinction. Calcium consumed as part of a regular diet appears to be handled differently by the body than calcium taken in tablet form. In particular, higher intake of calcium supplements has been associated with an increased risk of cardiovascular calcification and coronary heart disease, a risk that is not observed to the same degree with dietary calcium(36).

This difference points to a deeper principle. The body does not treat all nutrients equally simply because they are chemically similar. The way calcium is absorbed, distributed, and utilized depends on the context in which it enters the system.

Calcium obtained through food arrives gradually, accompanied by other minerals, vitamins, and cofactors that guide its metabolism. Supplements, on the other hand, deliver calcium in a concentrated form, often leading to a sudden rise in blood calcium levels. This abrupt increase appears to overwhelm the body's regulatory mechanisms, increasing the likelihood that calcium is deposited in places where it is not needed(37).

This brings us to an often-overlooked aspect of bone health: the role of use.

Bones are living tissues. They constantly remodel themselves in response to mechanical demand. When bones and joints are regularly loaded through movement, weight-bearing activity, and muscular engagement, the body receives a clear signal that structural strength is required. Under these conditions, calcium is directed toward the skeleton, where it contributes meaningfully to bone density and resilience(38)(23).

When this signal is absent, the situation changes. If a person is largely sedentary, avoids loading their joints, or does not challenge their skeletal system through movement, the body has little reason to increase bone hardness. In such cases, even if calcium is consumed in large amounts, the body may not incorporate it into bone tissue. Instead, calcium may remain in the bloodstream and is eventually excreted through the kidneys.

This process reflects what may be called body intelligence. The body does not strengthen structures that are not being used. Strength follows demand.

When excess calcium is not directed toward bone, it does not simply disappear. In some cases, it may deposit in soft tissues, including blood vessels. Calcification of the coronary arteries increases arterial stiffness and contributes to cardiovascular risk(37). This is one of the primary concerns raised in recent discussions about widespread calcium supplementation, especially in older adults.

Calcium supplementation after menopause has long been recommended to support bone health, given the accelerated bone loss associated with declining estrogen levels. However, contemporary evidence suggests that routine supplementation with calcium, with or without vitamin D, provides no clear net benefit for the primary prevention of fractures in otherwise healthy, community-dwelling postmenopausal women[39]. Large systematic reviews similarly report no consistent reduction in hip or overall fracture risk, indicating that supplementation should be viewed as one component of a broader approach to skeletal health rather than a standalone solution[40].

This does not mean that bone health is unimportant. On the contrary, it means that bone health cannot be reduced to a single nutrient.

Strengthening bones requires a combination of appropriate loading, muscular engagement, hormonal balance, adequate nutrition from whole foods, and nervous system regulation. Calcium plays a role, but it is not the driver. Movement is.

From a yogic and functional perspective, the most effective way to signal the body that stronger bones are required is through regular, intelligent use of the body. Weight-bearing postures, controlled loading of joints, and mindful movement provide the stimulus that supplements alone cannot replace.

Dietary sources of calcium, obtained through natural foods, integrate seamlessly into this process. They support bone health without overwhelming regulatory systems. Supplements, when used indiscriminately or in the absence of mechanical demand, may do more harm than good.

This is why caution is necessary. Taking calcium tablets without understanding whether they are needed, and without addressing movement and loading, may create a false sense of security. Bone strength cannot be swallowed. It must be earned through use.

The intention here is not to create fear around supplementation, nor to deny its role in specific clinical situations. There are cases where calcium supplementation is appropriate and medically indicated. However, routine and unnecessary use, especially as a substitute for movement and lifestyle change, deserves reconsideration.

The body responds intelligently when given the right signals. When we respect that intelligence, bone health becomes a natural outcome rather than a pharmaceutical goal.

# PAINKILLERS AND ANTI-INFLAMMATORY DRUGS

Painkillers and anti-inflammatory drugs are among the most commonly used responses to physical pain in modern healthcare. In some countries these are easily available as over the counter medicine without any prescriptions. For many people, they offer genuine and often immediate relief. Pain reduces, movement feels easier, and daily activities become manageable again. This relief can be deeply reassuring, especially when pain has been persistent or overwhelming. It is therefore understandable that pain reduction is often equated with healing.

Yet, in many cases, this equation is misleading. To understand why, it is important to distinguish clearly between pain reduction and functional recovery. Pain is not merely an unpleasant sensation to be removed. It is also a form of biological feedback. It reflects how tissues are being loaded, how movement is organized, and how the nervous system perceives safety or threat. When pain is chemically suppressed, this feedback system is altered. The signal becomes quieter, but the underlying pattern that produced the signal may remain unchanged.

Most commonly used painkillers work by altering either inflammatory processes or the way pain signals are processed by the nervous system. Non-steroidal anti-inflammatory drugs (NSAID) reduce chemical mediators associated with inflammation and sensitization. Other analgesics act centrally, dampening the perception of pain in the brain and spinal cord. What none of these interventions directly address is how the body is moving, how load is being distributed, or how coordination has adapted over time.

When pain reduces, people naturally return to activity. However, they usually return to activity using the same movement strategies that were present before the pain emerged. The difference now is that the protective warning system has been muted. Movements that were once limited by discomfort are performed more freely, but not necessarily more intelligently. Muscles that were overworking may continue to do so. Muscles that were inhibited may remain inactive. Joints may continue to receive uneven or excessive load. The absence of pain creates the impression that the system is functioning well, even when imbalance persists.

From a biomechanical perspective, pain reduction does not guarantee improved movement quality. It only changes perception. Coordination, stability, and load-sharing must be relearned through use, not assumed through symptom relief. This explains a pattern many people recognize: pain reduces with medication, activity increases, and after some time the pain returns. Sometimes it returns more intensely. Sometimes it appears in a different area altogether. The body has not healed. It has adapted further.

Pain also plays an important role in shaping movement behavior. When pain is present, the body naturally protects. Range of motion reduces, posture changes, and movement becomes cautious. These protective responses are not inherently harmful. They are intelligent short-term strategies. Problems arise when protection becomes chronic or unconscious. When pain is masked rather than understood, protective patterns persist without awareness. The person moves more, but moves poorly. Over time, this increases strain on tissues that were already vulnerable, often shifting the problem rather than resolving it.

Repeated or prolonged use of anti-inflammatory drugs also carries systemic consequences that are well documented in medical literature. These include irritation and ulceration of the gastrointestinal tract, increased risk of cardiovascular events, and impairment of kidney function. These are not rare or exceptional outcomes.

Large-scale clinical reviews and population studies support these concerns. Clinical guidelines and systematic analysis have consistently shown that while non-steroidal anti-inflammatory drugs are effective for short-term symptom control, they offer limited benefit for long-term functional recovery in chronic musculoskeletal pain conditions[27]. At the same time, extensive meta-analyses and re-evaluations of randomized trials have demonstrated a clear increase in gastrointestinal complications, cardiovascular events such as myocardial infarction and stroke, and renal impairment with prolonged or repeated NSAID use, even at commonly prescribed doses[41]. Gastrointestinal injury in particular has been shown to occur not only in high-risk individuals but also in otherwise healthy users, with risk increasing cumulatively over time[42].

Taken together, these findings suggest that while pain relief may be achieved, long-term reliance on anti-inflammatory medications often shifts the burden from localized pain to broader systemic risk without addressing the underlying drivers of dysfunction.

Beyond these systemic effects lies a more subtle issue that is rarely discussed. Healing is not simply the absence of pain. Healing is an adaptive process. Muscles strengthen in response to load and bones remodel according to use. The nervous system recalibrates through graded exposure, movement, and experience. When pain is consistently suppressed, the body receives fewer signals to reorganize itself. Instead of learning safer and more efficient ways to move, the system alternates between avoidance when pain is present and disregard when pain is absent. Neither state, fosters intelligent adaptation.

This does not mean that pain relief has no place in recovery. In acute injury, short-term pain control can reduce fear, prevent excessive guarding, and allow rest. It can create a window in which gentle movement, rehabilitation, and reorientation become possible. In such situations, pain relief supports healing rather than replacing it. The problem arises when medication becomes the primary or only response, without accompanying inquiry into posture, movement, and lifestyle.

Pain relief becomes particularly misleading when it creates the impression that nothing else needs to change. When posture remains unexamined, movement patterns remain inefficient, and daily habits remain unaltered, the absence of pain is temporary. The body continues to adapt beneath the surface. When medication is stopped, the system resumes signaling, often with greater urgency. This is not a failure of the body. It is a continuation of the same conversation that was interrupted rather than resolved.

From a yogic perspective, sustainable healing requires awareness rather than suppression. Pain is not treated as an enemy to be silenced, but as information to be interpreted. It points toward imbalance, overload, or loss of coordination. Pain relief can support this process, but it cannot substitute for it. When medication is used without reflection, it delays learning. When it is paired with movement awareness, education, and gradual re-engagement, it can play a constructive role within a broader healing process.

Painkillers and anti-inflammatory drugs are tools. Like all tools, their value lies in how they are used. When pain relief is combined with responsibility, patience, and appropriate movement, it may assist recovery. When it is used to bypass awareness or avoid engagement, it often prolongs the very problem it seeks to solve.

Healing is not achieved by removing discomfort alone. It emerges when the body is given the opportunity to relearn balance, coordination, and trust in movement. Pain relief may quiet the signal, but healing changes the system.

# MUSCLE RELAXANTS AND REST PRESCRIPTIONS

When pain does not subside quickly, one of the most common responses in clinical practice is the prescription of muscle relaxants along with advice to rest. At first glance, this approach appears sensible and compassionate. If muscles are tight and painful, relaxing them should reduce discomfort. If movement increases pain, resting the body should allow healing to occur. In acute situations, such as immediately after an injury or during a severe flare-up, this strategy can indeed provide short-term relief.

The problem arises when this approach becomes the primary or long-term solution.

Muscle relaxants work mainly by acting on the central nervous system rather than directly on the muscles themselves. They reduce the neural signals that maintain muscle tone, creating a generalized sense of looseness and calm. For many people, this leads to an immediate reduction in pain and a feeling that the problem is resolving. However, this relief often masks deeper issues related to coordination, movement patterns, and postural control.

To understand why these matters, we must first remember what muscles actually do. Muscles are not merely motors that contract and relax to produce movement. They are also sensory organs. Through constant communication with the nervous system, muscles provide feedback about position, movement, load, and balance. This internal sensing system is known as proprioception. It allows us to know where our body is in space without looking, to adjust posture automatically, and to distribute effort efficiently during movement.

When pain is present, proprioception, the body's ability to sense its position and movement, is often already altered. The nervous system becomes cautious, and movement may feel guarded or uncertain. Muscle relaxants further reduce this sensory feedback. While this can decrease the sensation of tightness and pain, it also interferes with the body's ability to sense itself accurately.

This can be understood through a simple analogy. Imagine trying to walk on uneven ground while wearing thick gloves on your feet. The ground is still there, but your ability to feel it is reduced. Because the brain is receiving unclear information about the surface, you may slow down, place your feet more carefully, lose balance more easily, or use excessive effort elsewhere to feel secure. The same thing happens internally when proprioceptive feedback is dampened. A similar effect can be noticed when walking in thick-soled footwear, where reduced sensory input alters balance and movement.

As proprioception decreases, coordination begins to suffer. Postural control becomes less precise. Movements that were already inefficient become more disorganized. The body, now operating with reduced internal feedback, often compensates in one of two ways. In some cases, it recruits other muscles excessively in an attempt to create stability. Muscles that were not meant to perform postural work become chronically overactive. This can lead to new areas of pain, fatigue, or stiffness. In other cases, the body limits movement altogether. Stiffness increases, and the person becomes hesitant to move, not because of pain alone, but because the body no longer feels safe or coordinated.

This explains a common clinical pattern. Many people report that muscle relaxants helped initially but later left them feeling weak, clumsy, heavy, or unstable. Some describe a loss of confidence in their movements. Others notice that pain has shifted to a different area of the body. The original pain may have reduced, but the system as a whole has become less organized.

Scientific literature supports these observations. Reviews of centrally acting muscle relaxants show that while they can reduce pain in the short term, their long-term benefits are limited. Prolonged use is associated with impaired motor control, reduced alertness, and increased risk of imbalance and falls, particularly when combined with inactivity[27][43].

The situation becomes more problematic when muscle relaxants are paired with prolonged rest.

Rest is often prescribed with the intention of protecting injured tissues. In the early stages of acute injury, short periods of rest can be helpful. However, extended rest reduces sensory input from muscles and joints even further. When movement decreases, the nervous system receives less information about alignment, load, and coordination. Muscles weaken, joints lose mobility and circulation reduces. The body's ability to organize itself efficiently declines.

Decades of research on back pain have shown that prolonged bed rest delays recovery rather than promoting it. Individuals who remain inactive for extended periods tend to experience greater stiffness, reduced strength, increased muscle weakness, and a higher risk of developing chronic pain. In contrast, early and graded movement has been consistently associated with better outcomes, improved function, and reduced recurrence of pain[44].

This highlights an important distinction that is often overlooked. Relaxation is not the same as inhibition. True relaxation occurs when the body feels coordinated, supported, and capable. Chemical relaxation suppresses muscle activity without restoring coordination. It quietens symptoms without teaching the body how to move better.

From a yogic perspective, healing occurs not by suppressing sensation, but by restoring communication within the system. Controlled movement, breath awareness, and gradual re-engagement of the body allow proprioception to return. Muscles relax not because they are chemically silenced, but because they no longer need to protect. Coordination improves. Confidence in movement grows. Pain reduces as a consequence, not as a target.

This does not mean that muscle relaxants and rest have no role. Short-term use during acute flare-ups can reduce suffering and create a window in which movement can be resumed more comfortably. The problem arises when they become substitutes for movement education instead of helping us start moving again.

The body heals through intelligent use, not prolonged avoidance. Rest without re-education leads to deconditioning. Relaxation without awareness leads to disorganization. Sustainable recovery emerges when clarity of movement is restored and the body is given the opportunity to relearn how to support itself.

PART V

# RECOGNIZING THE PATH TO RECOVERY

# SIGNS THAT HEALING IS POSSIBLE

After exploring the many dimensions of physical pain, a natural question arises. Is it possible to know whether back pain or neck pain can heal? Are there signs that indicate whether the body is capable of recovery without invasive intervention.

This question matters because not all pain arises from irreversible damage. Some pain reflects structural pathology that requires urgent medical care. Much of what people experience, however, belongs to a functional category, where the body has adapted to prolonged stress, altered movement, or protective patterns. Learning to recognize these distinctions reduces fear and helps prevent unnecessary escalation.

Several clinicians and physiotherapists have observed that certain patterns of pain strongly suggest a muscular, postural, or mechanical origin rather than permanent structural failure. These observations are supported by modern pain science, which emphasizes variability, adaptability, and context as key indicators of reversibility[(29)(28)].

One of the most important signs is the presence of pain-free moments during the day. Even if pain dominates much of the time, the ability to experience ten minutes without pain is significant. It indicates that the nervous system can down-regulate and that tissues are capable of resting and recalibrating. Research shows that fluctuating pain patterns are more commonly associated with functional pain states than with fixed structural damage, which tends to produce constant symptoms[(29)].

Modern pain science has shown that pain is not always a reliable indicator of tissue damage. In many cases, especially when pain persists long after tissues should have healed, the nervous system itself becomes overprotective. It begins to amplify signals of threat even in the absence of ongoing injury. This helps explain why pain can feel intense, widespread, or unpredictable despite normal imaging findings or minimal structural changes.

Research in pain neuroscience has demonstrated that factors such as fear, stress, prior experiences, and beliefs about the body can heighten the sensitivity of the nervous system, increasing pain perception without corresponding tissue harm[29][28]. In such situations, pain functions less as a signal of damage and more as a learned protective response.

When pain is maintained by nervous system sensitization rather than structural injury, it is often reversible without surgical intervention. Understanding pain in this way shifts the focus from fixing damaged parts to restoring a sense of safety in the body. Education, appropriate movement, and gradual re-engagement with activity help recalibrate the nervous system, allowing protection to soften and normal function to return[29][28].

Another important sign relates to posture and direction of movement. If bending forward increases pain, while straightening the body reduces it, this often reflects mechanical loading patterns rather than irreversible injury. This concept is well described in physiotherapy through the idea of directional preference, particularly within mechanical diagnosis frameworks such as the McKenzie Method[45]. When pain responds predictably to certain directions, it suggests that movement itself remains a useful therapeutic tool.

Pain that worsens with prolonged bending and twisting is another favorable indicator. Sustained flexion and rotational postures place cumulative stress on muscles, ligaments, and discs. Biomechanical studies have shown that repeated or prolonged loading, especially without adequate recovery, increases tissue strain even in healthy spines[46]. When pain arises under these conditions, it often reflects overload rather than damage, meaning that modifying how load is applied can lead to improvement.

Morning stiffness that improves after movement is another commonly observed sign. Pain that feels worse after rest and gradually eases once activity begins usually reflects tissue stiffness, reduced circulation, and protective muscle guarding rather than active injury[22]. Gentle movement restores fluid exchange, normalizes muscle tone, and improves joint mechanics, which is why pain often reduces once the body begins to move.

Closely related to this is pain that worsens with inactivity and improves with movement. Modern clinical guidelines consistently discourage prolonged bed rest for back pain, as inactivity has been shown to increase stiffness, weaken muscles, and prolong recovery[47]. When movement leads to relief rather than worsening, it strongly suggests that the body is seeking appropriate engagement rather than protection.

The location of pain also provides important information. Pain confined to the back or upper thigh, without radiating below the knee into the foot, is more often mechanical or muscular in origin. In contrast, true nerve root involvement typically presents with pain extending below the knee, often accompanied by neurological symptoms[25]. Localized pain patterns generally indicate a more favorable prognosis with conservative care.

Another encouraging sign is the ability to find relief in certain positions. If lying on the abdomen or gently extending the spine feels comfortable, it suggests tolerance to extension and responsiveness to positional change. Such responses are commonly used in physiotherapy assessments to identify mechanical pain patterns that respond well to guided movement[45].

Clinicians often observe that when multiple such signs are present together, the likelihood of improvement through non-invasive methods increases significantly. While no rigid numerical rule can predict recovery with certainty, research consistently shows that patients demonstrating several favorable mechanical indicators respond well to conservative treatment approaches such as Yoga therapy, exercise therapy, movement retraining, and education[47][48].

The essential requirement in such cases is regularity. Healing does not come from occasional effort or sporadic intervention. The body adapts to what it experiences repeatedly. Consistent, appropriately directed movement teaches tissues and the nervous system that activity is safe again. Early improvement may appear not as complete absence of pain, but as shorter pain duration, increased ease of movement, or longer pain-free intervals.

This framework is not meant to encourage self-diagnosis or delay necessary medical care. Rather, it supports informed decision-making. When the body shows signs of adaptability, conservative approaches deserve time, patience, and commitment.

In many cases, the body is not broken. It is responding intelligently to how it has been used, protected, or overloaded. When given the right inputs, it can relearn balance, strength, and ease of movement.

Healing, in such situations, is not a miracle. It is the gradual restoration of trust between the body and movement.

# WHY HEALING IS NOT LINEAR?

One of the most frustrating aspects of recovering from physical pain is the expectation that improvement should follow a straight line. We imagine healing as a steady progression: pain decreases, movement improves, and normal life resumes without interruption. When this does not happen, doubt sets in. A flare-up appears. Old symptoms return. Confidence collapses. Many people interpret this as failure or as proof that something is fundamentally wrong.

In reality, healing rarely unfolds in a straight line. Flare-ups during recovery are not signs that healing has stopped. They are often signs that the body is learning. As movement increases and old patterns begin to change, the nervous system is exposed to sensations it has not encountered in a long time. These sensations may feel unfamiliar or intense, even when they are not harmful. The nervous system, whose primary role is protection, may temporarily respond by increasing pain as a precaution.

This does not mean damage has occurred. It means the system is reassessing.

Early improvement often feels unstable because the body is transitioning from long-held compensations to new ways of moving. Muscles that were underused begin to work again. Joints that were protected regain motion. Sensory input increases. During this phase, the system has not yet established trust in these new patterns. It may fluctuate between the old habits and the emerging ones.

This is why someone may feel better one week and worse the next, even while doing everything "right." The system is reorganizing.

A useful distinction here is between adaptation and cure. Adaptation is the body's ability to adjust to circumstances. When pain first appears, the body adapts by stiffening, guarding, and limiting movement. These adaptations allow function to continue, but at a cost. Healing does not remove adaptation instantly. It replaces one form of adaptation with another.

Early in recovery, the body is adapting to movement rather than avoiding it. This new adaptation feels unfamiliar. It requires recalibration of strength, coordination, and confidence. Until this recalibration stabilizes, symptoms may fluctuate.

A cure implies an endpoint, a return to a previous state. Adaptation implies ongoing learning. The human body does not simply revert to an earlier version of itself. It evolves based on experience. Healing, therefore, is not about erasing pain, but about developing new capacities that make pain unnecessary.

From a yogic perspective, this process mirrors the nature of sadhana. Progress is not measured by the absence of obstacles, but by the quality of engagement. Fluctuations are expected. Awareness deepens gradually and stability emerges not through force, but through consistency.

When flare-ups are interpreted as danger, fear returns and avoidance resumes. When they are understood as part of the learning process, they lose their power. The body is allowed to continue to explore without retreat.

Healing feels unstable initially because stability is being rebuilt, not restored. The system is finding a new equilibrium, one that often differs from what existed before pain began. This new equilibrium is usually more resilient, more aware, and better coordinated.

Linear expectations create unnecessary suffering. When we accept healing as a dynamic process, patience replaces urgency. Confidence grows not because symptoms disappear permanently, but because the body demonstrates its ability to recover, adapt, and continue.

Healing is not a straight path. It is a conversation between effort and rest, movement and awareness, challenge and safety. When we listen carefully, the body shows us the way forward, even when the path curves.

# WHY EFFORT OFTEN DELAYS HEALING

When pain persists, the most natural response is to try harder: more exercises, stronger stretches, better posture, and greater discipline. Effort feels responsible and proactive, as if one is doing something rather than waiting helplessly. Yet, in the context of healing, especially from long-standing physical pain, effort can quietly become the very thing that delays recovery.

This is not because effort is wrong, but because effort is often misdirected. Many people approach rehabilitation with the same mindset they bring to fitness or achievement. They push through discomfort, repeat exercises aggressively, and measure progress by how much more they can do. When pain flares, they respond by adding more effort rather than changing quality. The body, however, does not interpret effort in the same way the mind does.

From the body's perspective, excessive effort often signals threat. When exercises are overdone, especially in the presence of pain, muscles tighten instead of coordinating. Breathing becomes shallow and movements lose fluidity. The nervous system shifts into a protective mode. What was intended as healing activity becomes another stressor that the system must guard against.

This is why people often say, "I am doing all the exercises, but my pain is not improving," or "I feel worse after trying to fix myself." The issue is rarely the exercise itself. It is the way the exercise is being performed and the internal state from which it is being approached.

> ***Always remember that it is not what we do but the way it is done matters.***

Forcing correction creates a similar problem. Posture, for example, is often treated as something to be held rather than something to emerge. People pull their shoulders back, tighten their abdomen, or rigidly straighten their spine in an attempt to maintain alignment. This effortful holding may look correct externally, but internally it increases tension and fatigue. The body is being controlled rather than reorganized.

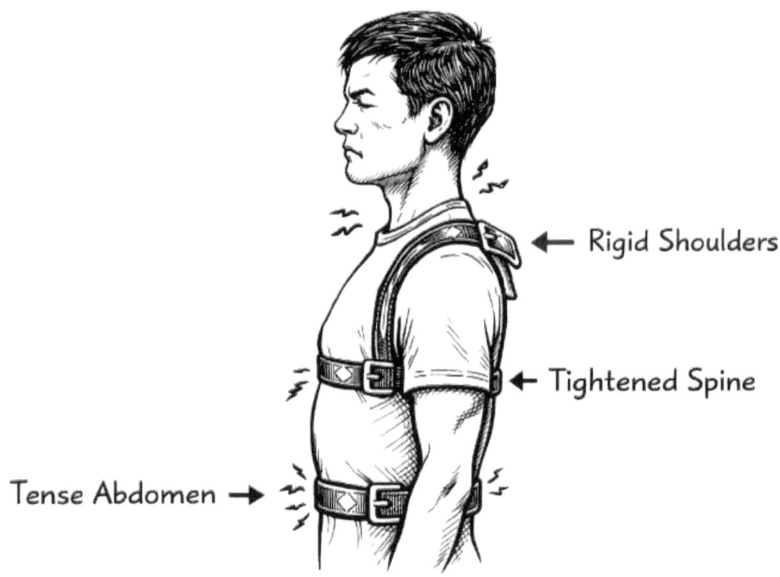


Increased Tension & Fatigue

True postural change does not come from holding the body in place. It comes from restoring balance, responsiveness, and ease. When alignment is forced, the system never learns how to support itself naturally. The moment attention drops, the body collapses back into old patterns, often with even more tension than before.

From a yogic perspective, this misunderstanding has been addressed for centuries through the principle of *sthira* and *sukha*, described in the Yoga

Sutras of Patañjali (2.46): स्थिरसुखमासनम् (sthira-sukham āsanam). *Sthira* conveys steadiness, stability, and supportive strength, while *sukha* denotes ease, comfort, and a sense of spaciousness. In classical Yoga, a posture is considered appropriate not because it appears perfect, but because it expresses both stability and ease at the same time.

Applied to rehabilitation, this principle becomes transformative. Healing emerges from a balance between effort that creates structure and ease that allows adaptation. Too little effort leads to no result and too much effort leads to guarding and resistance.

> ***The body heals in the narrow space where stability and comfort coexist.***

This balance is often counterintuitive for people in pain. When pain is present, the instinct is either to avoid movement completely or to attack the problem aggressively. Neither extreme allows the nervous system to feel safe. Safety is not created by intensity. It is created by predictability, gentleness, and clear feedback.

When movement is performed with excessive effort, the nervous system interprets it as strain. When movement is performed with awareness, controlled range, and steady breath, the nervous system receives a different message. It begins to understand that movement is possible without harm. Muscles relax not because they are forced to, but because they are no longer needed to protect.

This is why healing often accelerates when people do less, but do it better. Gentle movements done regularly are more effective than intense sessions done sporadically. Attention to breath restores rhythm and reduces unnecessary tension. Allowing the body to explore movement without judgment builds confidence. Over time, effort becomes more refined. Strength increases naturally. Pain reduces not because it was fought, but because it was no longer required as a warning.

Effort that delays healing is usually effort driven by fear, impatience, or control. Effort that supports healing is guided by listening, responsiveness, and respect for the body's pace.

In Yoga, this is not considered weakness. It is considered wisdom. Healing is not achieved by conquering the body. It unfolds when the body is allowed to reorganize itself under the right conditions. When steadiness is combined with ease, movement becomes restorative rather than demanding. Pain loses its purpose, and effort finally begins to work with the body instead of against it.

# TIME AS A THERAPEUTIC FACTOR

One of the most undervalued elements in healing is time. In a world trained to expect quick results, time is often seen as an obstacle rather than a resource. When pain persists beyond a few weeks, impatience sets in. Questions arise. Why is this not resolving? What else should I do? What intervention will fix this faster? Which doctor should I meet go fix it? In this climate, time is treated as a problem to overcome instead of a condition that allows healing to unfold.

> ***The body does not heal by intensity. It heals by consistency over time.***

Biological tissues follow their own rhythms. Muscles, tendons, ligaments, and connective tissue remodel gradually in response to repeated, appropriate loading. Nerves recalibrate sensitivity slowly through exposure and reassurance. These processes cannot be rushed without cost. Increasing intensity does not compress biological time. It often disrupts it.

This is why aggressive rehabilitation, despite good intentions, frequently leads to flare-ups. The tissues may not be injured, but they are not yet prepared. The nervous system may not be fragile, but it is not yet confident. Time allows adaptation to occur layer by layer. Intensity attempts to force change before the system is ready to receive it.

Impatience plays a powerful role in how people approach pain. When improvement is slow or uneven, doubt creeps in. The mind begins to question whether movement is enough, whether something is being missed, whether a stronger intervention is required. This psychological pressure often pushes people toward more invasive options, not because they are necessary, but because waiting feels intolerable.

Many medical interventions arise not from severity, but from urgency. This urgency is understandable. Pain disrupts life. It demands resolution. But when decisions are driven by impatience rather than understanding, the risk of overtreatment increases. Imaging is repeated. Procedures are escalated. Medications are intensified. The body is treated as something that needs to be fixed quickly rather than something that needs time to reorganize.

> ***Healing, however, is not a mechanical repair. It is a process of re-learning.***

The yogic tradition has articulated this truth with remarkable precision. Patañjali addresses the role of time in healing and transformation through a single sutra that remains profoundly relevant today.

**स तु दीर्घकालनैरन्तर्यसत्कारासेवितो दृढभूमिः॥**

*(Yoga Sūtra 1.14)*

sa tu dīrghakāla-nairantarya-satkārāsevito dṛḍhabhūmiḥ

Patañjali explains that any practice becomes firmly established only when it is undertaken over a long period of time (*dīrgha-kāla*), without interruption (*nirantarya*), and with complete devotion (*satkāra*). Only then does it reach *dṛḍha-bhūmiḥ*, a stable foundation that does not collapse under fluctuation.

This principle applies directly to healing. The body does not trust sudden change. It trusts what is consistent. Pain patterns dissolve not through dramatic effort, but through sustained, respectful engagement with movement and awareness. When practice is hurried, irregular, or driven by urgency, adaptation remains shallow. When it is patient, continuous, and kind, the nervous system gradually recalibrates, tissues reorganize, and confidence returns. Patañjali's insight reminds us time is the medium through which healing becomes real.

When pain has been present for a long time, the body has adapted. Muscles have learned to protect. Movement patterns have shifted. The nervous system has adjusted its thresholds. Healing does not erase these adaptations overnight. It replaces them gradually with new ones.

Re-learning requires repetition without threat. It requires exposure without fear. It requires time for the system to gather evidence that movement is safe again. Each pain-free or low-threat experience becomes a data point that slowly changes how the nervous system responds.

This is why early improvements often feel fragile. The new pattern is not yet dominant. The old one still exists. Time allows the balance to shift.

Time is not passive. It is active participation. Regular practice, even if gentle, creates continuity. Awareness deepens not through force, but through sustained attention. The body learns not because it is commanded to change, but because it is given repeated opportunities to respond differently.

> ***Fixing implies something is broken. Re-learning acknowledges intelligence.***

When healing is framed as fixing, impatience follows naturally. When healing is framed as learning, time becomes an ally rather than an enemy. Setbacks are understood as part of the process. Fluctuations are expected. Progress is measured not only by the absence of pain, but by increased confidence, ease, and adaptability.

The body remembers what it practices most. Time allows new experiences to outweigh old habits. It allows stability to emerge without rigidity and movement to return without fear.

Healing does not ask for urgency. It asks for presence. When time is respected as a therapeutic factor, the need for force diminishes. Interventions become more thoughtful. Effort becomes refined. And healing unfolds not as a sudden event, but as a quiet, cumulative transformation that lasts.

PART VI

# YOGA AS AN INTELLIGENT SUPPORT

# YOGA IS NOT EXERCISE: CALMING THE SYSTEM BEFORE CORRECTING THE BODY

For many people today, Yoga is understood primarily as a form of physical exercise. It is placed alongside stretching routines, fitness programs, or rehabilitation methods. In the context of back and neck pain, it is often approached as a way to loosen tight muscles, strengthen weak areas, or improve flexibility. While these effects can and do occur, they represent only a small portion of what Yoga truly offers[(49)].

In its classical understanding, Yoga was never defined as a physical workout. The foundational aphorism states: योगश्चित्तवृत्तिनिरोधः Yogaḥ cittavṛtti nirodhaḥ (Yoga Sutra 1.2)[(50)]. Yoga is the settling of the fluctuations of the mind. This definition shifts the center of attention immediately. The aim is not the muscle. It is not the joint. It is the state of the mind.

The physical practices were always secondary tools. They were designed to prepare the system for steadiness. Without that steadiness, even the most refined posture remains superficial. This distinction becomes crucial when we look at pain.

One of the consistent findings in both yogic insight and modern physiology is that pain is deeply influenced by the state of arousal within the nervous system[(51)]. When the mind is agitated or under sustained pressure, the sympathetic system becomes dominant. The body prepares for protection: muscle tone increases, breathing becomes shallow, and sensory vigilance heightens.

In the short term, this response is intelligent. It protects us. But when it persists, it quietly reshapes the body.

Muscles that are held in subtle contraction for long periods lose their capacity to fully relax. Circulation becomes less efficient, movements become guarded, and coordination becomes fragmented. What begins as protection gradually becomes discomfort, and over time, discomfort becomes pain.

This is why pain often intensifies during periods of emotional strain or sustained mental stress. The structure may not have changed, but the state has.

Conventional approach is often to correct posture by strengthening or stretching some muscles while the system remains highly reactive. Exercises are added, stretches are tried and strength routines are intensified. Yet, if the nervous system is still organized around vigilance, the body resists change. Effort increases without ease.

Yoga reverses this sequence. Before correcting the body, it calms the system. Through breath awareness, steady pacing, and internal attention, Yoga reduces unnecessary excitation. As the mind settles, muscle tone begins to soften naturally. This reduction is not imposed but emerges as the system begins to feel safer.

When the nervous system downshifts, the body becomes capable of learning again. Muscles begin to cooperate rather than compete, movements become smoother, and guarding decreases. Yoga does not force change but creates the conditions in which change becomes possible.

Seen this way, the asanas are not exercises in the conventional sense. They are conversations with the nervous system. Each movement communicates safety or urgency. Each pause communicates trust or control. The body listens.

When this communication becomes steady and respectful, the system reorganizes itself from within. Lasting change begins not with effort, but with regulation.

Understanding that regulation must precede correction raises a practical question. If calming the system is foundational, how exactly does one influence something as subtle as nervous system arousal? Muscles can be stretched. Postures can be adjusted but the state of the system itself requires a different entry point. Among all available tools, there is one that is immediate, accessible, and deeply transformative. That doorway is the breath.

# BREATH AS THE GATEWAY TO REGULATION

When the system remains in persistent activation, healing becomes difficult even in the absence of structural damage. The nervous system continues scanning for threat long after the original cause has resolved.

Before we attempt to change structure, we must understand how to change state.

From a yogic perspective, the most direct doorway into this shift is the breath.

Breath occupies a unique position in human physiology. It functions automatically, sustaining life without conscious effort. Yet it can also be consciously influenced. This dual nature makes it a bridge between voluntary awareness and the autonomic nervous system(52).

When sympathetic dominance prevails, breathing patterns alter: the breath becomes shallow and chest-oriented, exhalation shortens, and the rhythm becomes irregular. This pattern does not merely reflect stress but reinforces it.

This insight is not new. Classical yogic texts recognized the intimate relationship between breath and mind. The *Hatha Yoga Pradipika*(53) expresses this relationship with remarkable clarity:

चले वाते चले चित्तं निश्चले निश्चलं भवेत् ।
योगी स्थाणुत्वमाप्नोति ततो वायुं निरोधयेत् ॥

*(Hatha Yoga Pradipika 2.2)*

Chale vate chale chittam nischale nischalam bhavet
yogi sthanutvam apnoti tato vayum nirodhayet

When the breath moves, the mind moves.
When the breath becomes still, the mind becomes still.
By this steadiness, the yogi attains stability.
Therefore, the breath should be regulated.

This verse captures the essence of regulation. Breath and mind are not separate processes. They move together. When breath is agitated, the mind follows. When breath settles, the mind settles without force.

This is not poetic metaphor but a physiological truth. Shallow, irregular breathing continuously signals to the nervous system that the environment is unsafe or demanding. Muscles remain guarded and posture stays defensive. Even during moments of rest, the system does not fully downshift. The body may appear still, but internally it remains on alert.

This is why attempts to relax the body through effort alone often fail. Stretching tight muscles without addressing breathing patterns may provide temporary relief, but the body soon returns to its familiar state of holding. Regulation must occur at the level where mind and body intersect.

Breath provides this access. When breathing slows, deepens, and becomes more rhythmic, particularly when exhalation is allowed to lengthen naturally, the nervous system begins to receive a different message. Urgency diminishes and muscle tone gradually reduces. The body begins to experience safety from within rather than seeking it through control or avoidance.

This settling does not occur because the mind is instructed to be calm. It occurs because the breath becomes calm. As the Hatha Yoga Pradipika indicates, stillness of the mind follows stillness of the breath.

It is important to recognize and choose the breathing practices that are regulating. Techniques that emphasize force, intensity, or prolonged retention can increase arousal if introduced prematurely. When the system is already stabilized in excited state, adding further stimulation through the breath may deepen imbalance rather than resolve it.

Regulation begins by being aware of the breathing. Gentle, unforced breathing that restores continuity between inhalation and exhalation allows the system to relearn rest. The aim is not to manipulate the breath aggressively but to allow it to become steady.

Over time, this steadiness reduces baseline arousal. The abdomen softens and the rib cage becomes more mobile as the neck and back release habitual holding. Breath does not directly fix tissues but shifts the internal environment in which they exist.

In chronic pain, breath forms the foundation. Without regulation at this level, strengthening and stretching remain incomplete, but with it, the body becomes receptive, and breath becomes the gateway through which the system rediscovers safety.

As breathing becomes steady, the nervous system begins to downshift. But regulation alone is not the final step. The deeper transformation occurs when the body begins to reinterpret experience itself. When breath stabilizes, the system becomes receptive. It is then that movement, sensation, and posture can be re-examined not through fear, but through safety. To understand this shift more clearly, we must look at how the body moves from a state of threat to a state of inner stability.

# FROM THREAT TO SAFETY: HOW YOGA RESTORES INNER STABILITY

In the earlier chapters, we explored how the nervous system protects us. We saw that pain is not always a measure of damage, but often a measure of protection. We examined how prolonged activation can keep the body in readiness long after the original stress has passed. Muscle tone remains elevated. Movement becomes guarded. Relaxation feels unfamiliar.

What we must now understand is something more subtle. The nervous system does not organize itself around structure alone. It organizes itself around perceived safety.

Protection is triggered not only by injury, but by interpretation. When the system interprets a movement as risky, a posture as unstable, or a sensation as threatening, it responds accordingly. Muscle tone increases, breath changes, attention narrows, and pain may appear, not because tissues are failing, but because the system is attempting to prevent what it believes might happen.

In acute situations, this intelligence serves us well, but in persistent pain, the interpretation may remain long after the original cause has resolved. The body continues to behave as though danger is present, anticipating movements with caution, holding postures with subtle bracing, and preparing for impact even before bending or turning.

At this stage, the question is no longer only about structure. The deeper question becomes whether the body feels safe.

Safety is not created by explanation alone. Telling a person that their scan is normal may be helpful, but it does not automatically calm the system. Reassurance through words is useful, yet incomplete, because the nervous system updates itself through experience[54].

It must experience movement without escalation, load without collapse and sensation without injury. When such experiences accumulate, the system gradually revises its conclusions. This is where Yoga becomes deeply therapeutic.

Yoga does not impose rapid correction, rush range, or demand performance. Instead, it slows the process enough for the nervous system to observe without alarm. Movements are introduced gradually, transitions are deliberate, breath is continuous, and effort is moderated.

When movement unfolds slowly and breath remains steady, urgency reduces. With effort that is appropriate and not excessive, strain does not accumulate, and when attention stays present rather than reactive, anticipation softens.

Under these conditions, the meaning of movement begins to change.

A forward bend that once triggered guarding may begin to feel manageable. A rotation that once produced apprehension may become exploratory rather than defensive. The structure may not have changed dramatically, but the interpretation has.

Pain, seen in this light, functions as a protective boundary. When perceived threat decreases, the need for that boundary reduces. The system no longer signals with the same intensity because it no longer perceives the same level of risk.

This is why forceful stretching often aggravates symptoms. Force communicates urgency and speed communicates instability. Even with therapeutic intention, the nervous system registers intensity first, and if that intensity exceeds capacity, protective responses increase rather than decrease.[55].

Yoga communicates differently.

Rather than insisting on change, Yoga allows exploration, and instead of pushing the body into shape, it creates a space in which the body can reorganize itself. The breath becomes an anchor, the pace predictable, and effort measured.

With repetition, these experiences accumulate, and the nervous system begins to learn that movement does not automatically lead to harm. Muscle tone adjusts, not because it has been stretched away, but because it is no longer required at the same level. Guarding reduces, breath deepens without force, and the body regains responsiveness rather than remaining reactive.[(56)].

Safety does not mean passivity, and the body does not collapse into softness. Instead, it regains flexibility in its responses, with activation available when needed rather than constant, and stability achieved through coordination rather than bracing.

When this inner stability returns, healing becomes possible on multiple levels: neuroplastic adaptation improves, coordination retrains more efficiently, emotional reactivity softens, and structural corrections integrate without provoking resistance.

The movement from threat to safety is rarely dramatic. It is gradual. But it is foundational.

> ***Without safety, correction feels like effort.***
> ***With safety, reorganization becomes natural.***

In many cases, pain begins to lose its intensity not because it has been fought, but because it is no longer necessary.

# THE BODY LEARNS: NEUROPLASTICITY AND THE REWRITING OF PAIN

In the earlier chapters, we explored how pain is shaped not only by structure, but by protection. We saw that the nervous system learns from repeated experience. When movements are repeatedly associated with discomfort or threat, the system becomes vigilant, muscle tone increases, guarding becomes automatic, and anticipation begins even before action.

To understand how this pattern can change, we must look at a remarkable capacity of the human brain. That capacity is neuroplasticity.

Neuroplasticity refers to the brain's ability to reorganize itself in response to experience. The brain is not fixed. It does not operate through rigid wiring established once and for all. Instead, it continuously updates its internal maps based on what we repeatedly do, feel, and believe.

Within the brain are representations of the body and these are often referred to as body maps. Every movement of the neck, every shift in posture, every sensation from the lower back is interpreted through these maps. When movement is varied and confident, these maps remain clear and adaptable. When movement becomes limited, guarded, or fearful, the maps begin to change.

Chronic pain does not simply exist in tissues. It reshapes perception. When certain movements repeatedly trigger pain, the brain strengthens the pathways associated with those experiences[(51)]. The threshold for protection lowers. What once required significant stress to provoke discomfort may later require very little. The system becomes efficient at producing pain because it has learned that pain is necessary for protection.

This does not mean pain is imagined. It means pain is learned. Just as muscles adapt to repeated loading, neural pathways adapt to repeated signaling. The phrase by Donald O. Hebb, a Canadian psychologist, which says 'neurons that fire together wire together' captures this principle. When bending forward repeatedly triggers fear and discomfort, the brain begins to link forward bending with threat. Over time, the anticipation of bending may produce tension even before movement occurs.

This is known as fear-avoidance, which is not a sign of weakness but a form of protection shaped by repetition. When movement is avoided because it once caused pain, the brain receives fewer opportunities to update its conclusions, the body becomes less familiar with that movement, confidence decreases, and sensitivity increases. Avoidance reinforces the very pattern it seeks to prevent. In this way, chronic pain becomes partly a memory, with the body remembering what it believes to be dangerous.

The encouraging truth is that this process can work in both directions. If the nervous system can learn pain, it can also learn safety.

When movements are reintroduced slowly, deliberately, and without escalation, the brain receives new information. A forward bend performed with breath and control sends a different message than a rushed or forced movement. The system begins to observe that bending does not always result in harm. With repetition, this new association strengthens.

Neural pathways that once amplified protection begin to soften, body maps become clearer, movement feels less threatening, and the brain updates its expectations.

This is why slow repetition matters. Rapid or forceful movement often reinforces old patterns because the nervous system reacts quickly to intensity, and when speed exceeds the system's capacity, protection increases rather than decreases. Slow, mindful repetition allows the brain to remain engaged without becoming alarmed and creates space for perception to change[55].

In Yoga, repetition is not mechanical but attentive and explorative. Each movement is accompanied by awareness, each transition is observed, and breath remains continuous. This combination is intentional, precisely what supports adaptive neuroplasticity.

When breath remains steady during movement, the nervous system does not interpret effort as threat. When attention stays present, subtle improvements are noticed. Small successes accumulate and confidence grows quietly.

Over time, these repeated experiences reshape the internal landscape. Pain may not disappear overnight, but its intensity and frequency begin to shift. Movements that once felt guarded begin to feel accessible. Postures that once provoked apprehension become neutral. This transformation is rarely dramatic. It is gradual, layered, and cumulative. But it is real[56].

Neuroplasticity also connects directly to stabilization of arousal. When the system has been living at an elevated baseline of activation, the brain has adapted to that level of vigilance. Through deeper breath, right pacing, and mindful repetition, Yoga lowers this baseline gradually. As arousal stabilizes at a calmer level, new neural patterns become possible.

The body begins to move without bracing, the mind observes without anticipating danger, and protection becomes flexible rather than rigid.

This is not about forcing positive thinking or overriding pain signals. It is about providing consistent experiences that contradict outdated assumptions. When the system repeatedly experiences movement without harm, it rewrites its internal predictions.

In this sense, Yoga is not merely stretching or strengthening. It is participation in the brain's learning process. Each practice session becomes an opportunity to refine perception. Each breath becomes a signal of safety and each mindful repetition becomes a step in reorganizing the relationship between sensation and threat.

> ***The body learns through experience, and when experience changes, learning changes.***

Pain that was once entrenched can become less convincing. Guarding that once felt automatic can become optional. The system that once overprotected can regain discrimination.

Healing, then, is not only structural or muscular. It is neurological. It is the gradual rewriting of patterns that were once necessary but are no longer required.

And when the brain updates its maps, the body follows.

# MOVEMENT THAT RE-EDUCATES THE BODY

In the previous chapter, we explored how pain reshapes neural pathways and how the brain updates its maps through repeated experience. If pain can be learned, safety can also be learned. Movement is one of the primary ways this learning occurs.

But not all movement teaches the same lesson.

In many conventional approaches, movement is prescribed to strengthen, stretch, or increase endurance. The focus is often on output, repetition, and measurable progress. While such approaches can improve performance, they do not always address how the body organizes itself during movement. In the context of chronic back and neck pain, this difference becomes crucial.

Pain is rarely the result of weakness alone and more often reflects poor coordination. Some muscles work excessively while others remain underused, causing movements to be uneven. Certain segments of the spine carry more load than intended, while others remain stiff or disengaged. Over time, this imbalance overloads specific tissues and reinforces protective patterns[(55)].

If neuroplasticity tells us that the brain rewires through repetition, then the quality of repetition matters. Movement can either reinforce guarding or retrain coordination[(33)].

Yoga approaches movement as education rather than conditioning. Every asana, every transition, and every pause becomes an opportunity to refine internal communication. Instead of isolating a muscle or forcing a range, Yoga invites integration. The feet inform the pelvis, the pelvis supports the spine, the spine organizes the rib cage, and the breath links them all. Nothing functions independently.

This whole-body participation reduces unnecessary compensation. A muscle that was once in spasm may soften not because it was aggressively stretched, but because it is no longer required to perform the work of another region. When roles are clarified, effort distributes more evenly.

Range of motion develops in this context as well. Flexibility is not pursued as an isolated goal. It emerges as coordination improves and perceived threat reduces. When the nervous system feels safe and muscles coordinates better, joints begin to move more freely. This freedom is stable because it is supported by integration rather than force.

Strength, too, is redefined. Instead of pushing muscles to fatigue, Yoga builds strength through precise engagement and sustained attention. Muscles learn to support joints intelligently. Particularly in the spine, where excessive effort can aggravate symptoms, this kind of intelligent strength is essential. Stability arises from cooperation, not bracing(57).

Attention plays a central role in this retraining process. In many physical activities, attention is directed outward toward goals or performance, but in Yoga, it turns inward. Sensation becomes the guide, and subtle shifts in weight, breath, and effort are observed. This inward attention refines proprioception, the body's sense of position and movement.(16).

As proprioception improves, confidence improves. Movements that once felt threatening become predictable. Guarding reduces. The system no longer prepares for impact before every bend or turn. In this way, movement becomes a corrective experience for the brain's body maps.

Yoga also respects variability. What matters is not how a shape looks, but how it is experienced. Because pain arises from different patterns in different individuals, movement must remain adaptable. The same forward bend may need to be approached differently on different days. This responsiveness prevents repetition from becoming mechanical.

> ***Mechanical repetition reinforces old patterns, whereas mindful repetition rewrites them.***

Through consistent, attentive practice, the body begins to reorganize itself. Muscles coordinate more efficiently. Joints regain trust in movement. The spine no longer feels like a fragile structure requiring protection at every step. It becomes a dynamic conduit for force and expression.

Pain diminishes not because it is suppressed, but because the system no longer interprets movement as dangerous. Neural pathways that once amplified protection are gradually replaced by pathways that support confidence.

In this way, Yoga does not exhaust the body. It educates it. It does not impose change from the outside. It creates conditions in which the brain and body can update themselves from within.

As this retraining unfolds, movement becomes lighter. Posture organizes itself with less conscious effort. Daily activities begin to feel less like threats and more like expressions of capacity.

The body learns. And through intelligent movement, it learns differently.

# YOGA AND THE REDISTRIBUTION OF FORCE

In the previous chapter, we explored movement as neural retraining. We saw that Yoga educates coordination rather than exhausting muscles. When coordination improves, the brain updates its maps and guarding begins to reduce.

There is another layer to this learning. As we have learnt earlier, pain always appears in the weakest link in the body. When one region repeatedly absorbs more load than it is prepared to handle, protection increases and symptoms emerge. If movement retrains the nervous system, it also retrains how force travels through the body[57][55].

Yoga does not attempt to fix one painful segment in isolation. Instead, it improves how the entire system participates in sharing load.

In a simple standing posture practiced with awareness, weight begins to spread more evenly through the feet. The arches respond, the knees align more naturally, the pelvis adjusts subtly, the spine organizes itself without being forced upright, and the head balances rather than being held in place. Nothing dramatic occurs, yet gravity is distributed differently.

Balancing asanas refine this process further. The center of gravity becomes immediately relevant. The body cannot rely on rigid bracing. It must make continuous micro-adjustments. Muscles engage and release in coordination. Stability arises through responsiveness rather than stiffness.

Similarly in forward bending asanas, intelligent practice ensures that load is shared between hips and spine. The lumbar region is no longer forced to perform all the movement. The hips contribute. The posterior chain gradually adapts. The spine flexes with support rather than collapse.

Gentle backbends return extension to regions that have long remained flexed through habitual sitting. The thoracic spine begins to participate again. As mobility is restored above, the neck is relieved of compensating for what the mid-back cannot provide.

Twisting postures distribute rotation across multiple segments. Instead of concentrating torque at one vulnerable level, movement is shared. Each region contributes within its capacity.

Even transitions become meaningful. Rising from the floor, shifting weight, turning, and stabilizing are no longer casual actions. They become opportunities to practice balanced effort. The system learns that load can move through it without overwhelming any single point.

Gradually, the weak link is no longer overburdened. The lower back does not need to compensate for stiff hips. The neck does not need to carry the consequences of a collapsed thoracic spine. The shoulders do not brace for an unstable trunk(57). Force begins to travel more evenly.

This redistribution is not achieved through intensity. It develops through repetition with awareness. As coordination improves, muscles assume their appropriate roles. Fascia adapts to more balanced tension. Joints move within ranges that feel stable rather than strained.

Pain often reduces not because the painful area was attacked directly, but because it is no longer asked to do more than its share(55).

> ***When force is shared, strain decreases, protection lessens, and pain often softens.***

Yoga, in this sense, is not correcting posture in a cosmetic way. It is improving participation. Each region of the body contributes appropriately.

No segment is left isolated. No area is forced to carry disproportionate responsibility.

Postures become laboratories for force management. They are places where gravity is negotiated intelligently rather than resisted.

As the body relearns how to share load, it also relearns something essential: trust.

# YOGA THERAPY IS NOT ASANA THERAPY

At this point, it becomes necessary to clarify something that is often misunderstood.

When people hear that Yoga can help with back or neck pain, they usually think of postures. They imagine specific stretches for the lower back, strengthening poses for the shoulders, or alignment corrections for the neck. In many modern settings, Yoga is presented almost entirely through the lens of asana.

But Yoga therapy is not the same as asana therapy.

Asana is one limb within a much broader framework. Classical Yoga describes an eightfold path that includes not only posture, but also self-regulation, discipline, breath refinement, sensory management, concentration, and meditation (Yoga Sutra 2.29)[(50)]. When we reduce Yoga to asanas or posture alone, we narrow a systemic approach into a local intervention.

Back and neck pain do not arise from muscles alone. Earlier in this book, we explored how pain is influenced by nervous system sensitivity, patterns of protection, breathing habits, emotional load, and lifestyle demands. If the origin of strain is distributed across multiple dimensions, then an approach limited to posture cannot fully address it[(58)].

The broader vision of Yoga is beautifully expressed in the Bhagavad Gita 6.17:

युक्ताहारविहारस्य युक्तचेष्टस्य कर्मसु ।
युक्तस्वप्नावबोधस्य योगो भवति दुःखहा ॥

*yuktāhāra-vihārasya yukta-cheṣhṭasya karmasu*
*yukta-svapnāvabodhasya yogo bhavati duḥkha-hā*

For one who is moderate in food and recreation, balanced in action, regulated in sleep and wakefulness, Yoga becomes the destroyer of sorrow.

This verse widens the picture immediately. Yoga is not presented as a posture routine. It is presented as balance in living. Moderation in eating. Regulation in activity. Harmony between effort and rest. Stability in daily rhythm.

When this balance is absent, strain accumulates. When daily habits swing between excess and neglect, the body reflects that imbalance. The spine, constantly negotiating gravity and effort, becomes a visible site where this dysregulation expresses itself[59].

Asana can certainly improve coordination and help redistribute load. It can restore mobility where stiffness has accumulated. But if the internal state remains restless, if sleep is disturbed, if effort is excessive, or if daily activity lacks moderation, posture practice alone cannot resolve the deeper pattern.

Yoga therapy therefore includes more than shapes.

Breath is not an accessory to movement. It shapes internal rhythm and influences how the body responds to demand. Awareness is not decorative instruction. It determines whether movement becomes mechanical repetition or meaningful reorganization. Discipline is not rigid control but is steady alignment with what supports balance[60].

Lifestyle becomes part of therapy. The way one sits, works, responds to stress, and alternates between activity and rest directly influences spinal health in particular and our overall health in general. Without addressing these patterns, therapeutic gains remain fragile.

Even foundational principles such as non-harm and moderation have physical consequences. When effort is excessive, muscles tighten defensively. When discipline becomes harsh, the nervous system remains vigilant. When practice becomes competitive, protection increases rather than decreases.

Yoga therapy, therefore, does not treat the spine as an isolated structure. It considers the rhythms of living that shape the spine every day.

Meditation also plays its role. When the mind becomes less reactive, muscular tone adjusts accordingly. Posture becomes less about holding and more about balancing. Effort becomes appropriate rather than excessive.

Seen in this light, Yoga therapy does not aim to fix one segment of the body. It supports the person as a whole system.

Asana remains valuable. It is a powerful and practical doorway. But without the support of breath, awareness, behavioral balance, and disciplined living, posture practice becomes another mechanical intervention applied to a complex organism.

When this broader understanding is preserved, Yoga therapy regains its integrity. It becomes not merely a set of corrective techniques, but a way of living that gradually reduces suffering at its roots.

# THE EIGHT LIMBS OF YOGA AND THE HEALING OF PAIN

If we step back and look at everything we have discussed so far, one truth becomes clear.

Pain is not only biomechanical.

It is not only muscular.

It is not only structural.

It is layered.

It involves posture and gravity.

It involves coordination and force distribution.

It involves the nervous system and its perception of threat.

It involves habits, memory, emotion, and interpretation.

If pain arises across layers, healing must also move across layers.

This is where the classical framework of Ashtanga Yoga becomes deeply relevant. The eight limbs described by Patañjali for beginners are not merely philosophical ideals (Patañjali Yoga Sutra 2.29)[(50)]. They outline a progressive organization of human functioning, moving from behavior and lifestyle to body, breath, attention, and eventually taking one towards the ultimate goal of life which is liberation or Samadhi.

Seen through this lens, the eight limbs offer a comprehensive framework for understanding how healing can unfold.

## Yama - Reducing Inner Violence

The first step toward healing begins with relationship.

Many people approach their bodies with impatience, frustration, or force. They push into pain, override fatigue, or criticize themselves for limitations. This subtle aggression increases guarding. When the body is treated as an opponent, it responds protectively. Muscle tone rises, breath becomes shallow and movement becomes defensive.

However, concept of Ahimsa or non-violence, introduces a different approach. Effort becomes respectful when sensation is listened to rather than overridden. The body begins to experience cooperation rather than conflict.

Similarly, truthfulness also plays a role. Acknowledging fatigue, recognizing stress, and accepting present capacity create the conditions for intelligent progress. When honesty replaces denial, effort becomes appropriate. Remember that reducing internal conflict reduces unnecessary tension.

## Niyama - Inner Discipline

Healing does not occur through occasional effort. It requires daily practice and repetitions.

Irregular sleep, chaotic schedules, and inconsistent practice disturb nervous system stability. Whereas consistency supports regulation. When daily rhythms become predictable, the system expends less energy maintaining vigilance. This is where having a proper daily routine for every activity we do is extremely important to create a predictable system within us.

Not being content with our efforts will make us push our-self more which results in guarding. Contentment reduces the constant striving that keeps the body in readiness. Acceptance of our limitation and capabilities allows gradual progress.

Disciplined effort supports neuroplastic change. The body reorganizes through repetition, not intensity. Self-study deepens awareness of patterns: how one sits, or stands, breathes under stress, or responds to discomfort. Without this awareness, habits repeat automatically.

A willingness to release excessive control is equally important. Many chronic pain states are sustained by constant internal struggle. When effort softens and control reduces, the system becomes less guarded.

## Asana - Stability and Ease

Asana is described as something that is steady and comfortable. This definition is particularly relevant in the context of spinal issues. As we have discussed earlier stability does not mean rigidity and ease does not mean collapse.

When posture is approached with this understanding, load begins to distribute more evenly. Overactive regions soften and underused regions participate. The spine then begins to share load more intelligently.

Asanas are not some postures to achieve but are opportunities to experience and find balance. When balance improves, effort reduces.

## Pranayama - Regulation of Arousal

As we have explained earlier, breathing patterns both reflect and influence nervous system activity. When breath becomes shallow and rapid, vigilance increases. When breathing becomes smooth and continuous, urgency reduces. Pranayama develops this continuity. The breath lengthens naturally, and rhythm stabilizes.

As the internal environment becomes calmer, muscle tone reduces and protective guarding softens. Pain often becomes less intense when the system no longer perceives constant urgency. The breath alters the baseline from which the body operates.

## Pratyahara - Reducing Overstimulation

Modern life exposes the nervous system to continuous input. Screens, noise, and constant information maintain a background of alertness. The system rarely experiences withdrawal from stimulation.

Pratyahara involves reducing unnecessary sensory load. This does not mean withdrawing from life but instead it means allowing periods of quiet in which the nervous system can settle. When overstimulation reduces, internal sensitivity stabilizes and the body no longer scans constantly for threat. Eventually subtle muscular holding decreases.

## Dharana or Retraining Attention and Focus

Pain narrows attention as the mind anticipates discomfort and remains fixed on the affected area. This anticipation amplifies protective responses, and focused attention helps retrain this pattern. When awareness can rest on breath, alignment, or movement without panic then attention becomes deliberate rather than reactive.

This shift influences neural organization, as brain maps reorganize through repeated experience. When attention stabilizes without fear, perception changes and movement begins to feel manageable rather than threatening.

## Dhyana - Continuity of Regulation

When attention becomes steady and effortless, regulation becomes continuous. Reactivity reduces, emotional responses soften and guarding decreases.

Pain may still arise, but it is experienced differently. Sensation can be observed without immediate alarm, the nervous system no longer escalates every signal, and the system gradually becomes less defensive and more adaptable.

## Samadhi - Freedom from Identification with Pain

At the deepest level, suffering is intensified when one identifies with pain. When a person begins to believe they are fragile or permanently damaged, it reinforces guarding. The nervous system continues to protect against anticipated harm.

As identification loosens, the relationship with pain changes. Sensation may still arise, but it no longer defines the individual. This shift does not deny physical experience but it reduces the emotional burden attached to it. Freedom begins not in the spine alone, but in perception.

Seen together, the eight limbs describe a comprehensive process. Pain is not addressed at a single level. It is approached as a whole-system experience. When Yoga is understood in this integrated way, therapy is no longer limited to muscles and joints. It becomes a process of restoring balance across the entire human system. And as balance returns across these layers, the body often begins to do what it has always been capable of doing. It reorganizes.

# PAIN FROM THE PANCHAKOSHA PERSPECTIVE

Up to this point, we have explored pain through several lenses. We have examined the structure of the spine, the role of muscles and connective tissues, the influence of the nervous system, the impact of lifestyle habits, and the ways in which Yoga can restore coordination and stability.

Each of these perspectives helps explain part of the experience of pain. Yet the human system is more complex than any single explanation can capture. Physical discomfort is rarely confined to muscles or joints alone. Classical Yoga has long recognized this complexity.

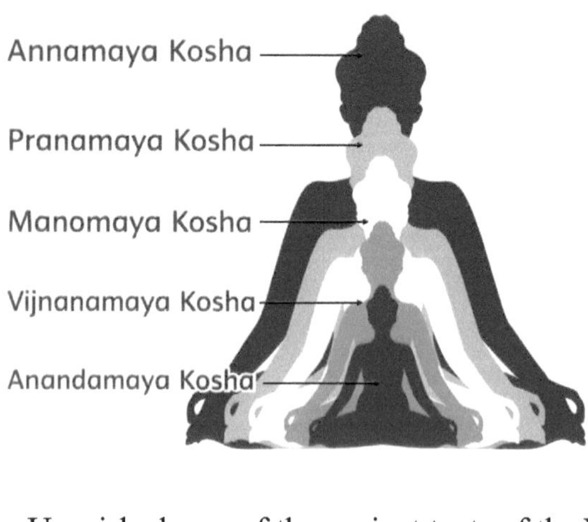


In the Taittiriya Upanishad, one of the ancient texts of the Yogic tradition, the human being is described as consisting of several interconnected layers known as the Panchakosha, or the five sheaths of existence. These sheaths are not separate bodies stacked one inside another. Rather, they represent different dimensions of the same living system, each influencing the others continuously.

Understanding this model can help us appreciate why pain sometimes persists even when structural damage is minimal, and why healing often requires attention to more than the physical body alone.

## The Physical Layer: Annamaya Kosha

The outermost layer is the Annamaya Kosha, often described as the physical body.

This is the body made of tissues, bones, muscles, ligaments, tendons, and organs. It is nourished by food, shaped by movement, and influenced by the environment in which we live. Most discussions about back and neck pain focus primarily on this level. Attention is directed toward discs, joints, muscles, and posture. Treatments often attempt to strengthen certain areas, stretch others, or correct alignment.

These approaches are important. The physical body must function well for the spine to remain healthy. However, as we have already seen, structural explanations alone cannot fully account for the experience of pain. As seen earlier, two people may show similar findings on an imaging scan, yet one may experience significant pain while the other feels none. This observation reminds us that the physical body is only one part of a larger system.

## The Energy Layer: Pranamaya Kosha

The next layer is the Pranamaya Kosha, the sheath associated with vital energy.

In modern physiological language, this layer can be understood through processes or functions such as breathing patterns, circulation and autonomic nervous system regulation. Breath has a direct influence on the state of the nervous system. As we have discussed in the earlier chapter on breath, when breathing becomes shallow and irregular, the body tends to remain in a state of vigilance. Muscles stay guarded, and relaxation becomes difficult.

Many individuals living with chronic pain also show disturbed breathing patterns. The breath may remain confined to the upper chest, exhalation may be shortened, and pauses in breathing may disappear. They continuously signal urgency to the nervous system.

Yoga recognizes breath through Pranayama practices, as a powerful gateway for restoring balance in this layer. When breathing becomes slower, deeper, and more rhythmic, the body begins to experience safety. Muscle tone reduces, circulation improves, and the nervous system gradually settles.

In this way, working with breath influences pain even though no direct mechanical intervention is applied to the spine.

## The Mental and Emotional Layer: Manomaya Kosha

Beyond the breath lies the Manomaya Kosha, the layer associated with thoughts, emotions, and sensory processing.

Pain is deeply influenced by this level. Fear, anxiety, frustration, and persistent mental stress can amplify the body's protective responses. The nervous system becomes more sensitive, and movements that were once neutral may begin to feel threatening.

This does not mean that pain is imaginary or purely psychological. Rather, it reflects the reality that the mind and body function as a unified system. Emotional states influence breathing, muscle tone, and attention. In turn, these changes affect how pain is perceived. For example, when a person becomes anxious about a particular movement, the body often tightens even before the movement begins. Muscles brace in anticipation of harm. Over time, this anticipation can reinforce pain patterns.

Yoga practices that cultivate awareness, and relaxation through various meditation, help calm this layer of the system. As mental agitation reduces, the body often releases unnecessary holding.

## The Layer of Understanding: Vijnanamaya Kosha

The fourth layer is the Vijnanamaya Kosha, sometimes described as the sheath of discernment or understanding.

This layer relates to how we interpret our experiences. Beliefs about the body, expectations about pain, and the meaning we attach to symptoms all influence how the nervous system responds. For example, if someone believes that a disc bulge means their spine is permanently fragile, they may begin to avoid many normal movements. This avoidance reduces activity, weakens muscles, and increases sensitivity. Over time, fear itself becomes a contributor to persistent pain.

On the other hand, when individuals understand that many spinal changes are part of natural adaptation and that the body retains the capacity to reorganize, their relationship with movement changes and confidence gradually returns.

Education therefore becomes therapeutic. When understanding deepens, the nervous system receives new information about safety and possibility. This book in in fact an attempt to influence at this level.

## The Innermost Layer of Ease: Anandamaya Kosha

The innermost layer described in the Panchakosha model is the Anandamaya Kosha, the sheath associated with inner ease and well-being.

This level is not about constant happiness or the absence of challenge. Rather, it reflects a deeper sense of steadiness and acceptance within the individual. When people live in persistent discomfort, their relationship with the body often becomes strained. The body may feel like an adversary rather than an ally. This tension can further reinforce stress and vigilance.

Yoga invites a gradual shift in this relationship. Through awareness, breath, movement, and reflection, individuals begin to reconnect with a sense of trust in their own bodies. Pain may still arise at times, but it is no longer interpreted as a catastrophe. This change in relationship can be profoundly healing.

The Panchakosha model reminds us that pain rarely belongs to only one layer of our being. A tight muscle may be influenced by breathing patterns. Breathing may be influenced by emotional stress. Emotional stress may be shaped by beliefs about the body. Beliefs may shift when understanding deepens. Each layer interacts with the others continuously.

Yoga therefore approaches healing as a process that includes the body, breath, mind, understanding, and inner orientation. Physical practices such as asana are important, but they are only one doorway into this larger system. When multiple layers begin to reorganize together, change becomes more stable and sustainable.

Pain that once seemed stubborn may begin to soften, not because one structure has been forced into correction, but because the entire system has gradually returned toward balance.

# RESTORING FLOW AND THE CONDITIONS FOR HEALING

When pain persists, it is rarely because the body lacks effort. More often, it is because something essential is not flowing. Traditional Yoga describes this disruption in terms of prana, the organizing force that governs movement, sensation, repair, and regulation. Modern physiology describes similar processes through blood flow, neural signaling, lymphatic movement, hormonal balance, and tissue hydration. Though the language differs, the observation is the same. Where there is rigidity or excessive holding, healing becomes difficult. Healing depends on circulation, communication, and coordination. When these processes are disturbed, recovery slows, even when structures appear intact.

Painful areas are almost always areas of holding. A muscle in spasm is not simply tight but is guarded. It behaves as if movement is unsafe. Circulation reduces, sensory feedback becomes less clear, and the nervous system begins to treat the region as a zone of threat. Even after tissues have healed structurally, this guarded state can persist, sustaining the experience of pain(55).

> ***Yoga does not attempt to force release. Instead, it restores flow gradually and intelligently.***

Gentle, coordinated movement changes the internal environment of tissues. Circulation improves, temperature normalizes, sensory input becomes clearer, and the nervous system updates its assessment of safety. As these experiences accumulate, protective tension is no longer required and release occurs as a consequence rather than an objective(61).

Breath supports this process, not as a technique to control, but as an organizing rhythm. When movement follows the rhythm of breathing rather than competing with it, effort becomes efficient and internal conflict reduces[(52)]. The body experiences continuity rather than fragmentation.

Equally important is rest. Modern culture often equates healing with action: more exercises, more repetitions, more intervention. Yet, healing requires periods of integration. Without adequate rest, the nervous system remains overstimulated, even when activity appears gentle.

Yoga recognizes the necessity of both stimulation and assimilation. Periods of effort are followed by periods of quiet integration. During these intervals, the nervous system recalibrates, muscles reorganize, and patterns learned during movement are absorbed rather than overwritten by fatigue.

This balance between effort and ease is described in yogic thought as sthira and sukha: stability without rigidity, ease without collapse (Patañjali Yoga Sutras 2.46)[(50)]. Flow is influenced not only by physical factors but also by emotional holding. Unresolved stress or fear can maintain muscular guarding long after the original trigger has passed. When physical flow is restored, emotional regulation often improves simultaneously, even without deliberate psychological processing.

As flow returns across multiple levels, physical symptoms begin to change. Pain becomes less intense, less frequent, and less alarming. Movement feels safer and the body regains confidence. Sensation becomes information rather than threat.

# WHY YOGA PRACTICE CANNOT BE PRESCRIBED

After understanding the anatomy, biomechanics, responses of the nervous system, emotional influences, and adaptive nature of pain, an important realization emerges. Healing cannot be reduced to a formula. Consequently, Yoga practices cannot be standardised.

This is where many misunderstandings about Yoga begin.

Modern healthcare often works through protocols. A diagnosis is followed by a set of recommended interventions. While this approach is effective for many acute and clearly defined conditions, it becomes limited when applied to chronic pain, postural dysfunction, and long-standing movement adaptations. These conditions are not static problems but are dynamic processes shaped by how the body has learned to respond over time.

Yoga does not operate as a prescriptive science because the human system it works with is not uniform. Two individuals may arrive with the same medical diagnosis, similar imaging findings, and comparable pain levels, yet require entirely different approaches. One person may be held in fear, guardedness, and excessive muscle tone and another may be collapsed, deconditioned, and disconnected from sensation. Applying the same practice to both would ignore the very intelligence Yoga seeks to honor.

Even within the same individual, the body's needs are not constant. What supports healing at one stage may become inappropriate at another. A practice that brings relief early on may later require refinement, progression, or even reduction. As the body changes, capacity evolves and sensitivity shifts, and static prescriptions fail to account for this living process.

This is why Yoga, in its therapeutic application, is always contextual. A meaningful practice considers posture, movement history, breath patterns, emotional state, energy levels, and the person's relationship with pain itself. It observes not only what the body can do, but how it does it. Is there strain? Is there holding? Is there hesitation or force? These subtle qualities matter as much as visible alignment.

This also explains why Yoga practices cannot be fully transmitted through books or videos. While education builds understanding, practice requires feedback. An experienced teacher does not merely instruct asanas. They observe effort, breath continuity, facial tension, transitions, and recovery. These observations guide real-time adjustments that prevent overdoing and support integration. Without this feedback loop, well-intentioned practice can unintentionally reinforce the very patterns it aims to undo.

Equally important is the recognition that pain does not always originate at the physical level. There are times when movement alone is not enough. Emotional strain, unresolved stress, mental fatigue, or long-standing psychological patterns may be contributing to physical symptoms. Yoga addresses these dimensions through its comprehensive Ashtanga Yoga system, and, at times, simple human conversation. These elements cannot be standardized or rushed. They require presence, trust, and sensitivity.

In this sense, Yoga is not a technique applied to the body. It is a relationship cultivated with the system as a whole.

Healing then becomes less about fixing something that is broken and more about restoring communication. It involves learning how much effort is appropriate, when to pause, and when to challenge or soften. This discernment grows through consistent, attentive practice rather than forceful intervention.

Throughout this book, the intention has not been to provide ready-made solutions or universal practices. Techniques without context can easily become mechanical. Instead, it has been to offer clarity. To help you understand why pain behaves the way it does. Why quick fixes often fail. Why the body responds not just to what we do, but to how we do it.

When Yoga is approached as a living process rather than a set of exercises, it supports change across physical, emotional, and neurological dimensions. It does not promise instant relief, but it offers something more valuable: a way to listen, a way to adapt, and a way to participate consciously in one's own healing.

If this book has tried to achieve anything, is the shift in perspective. Pain is no longer an enemy to be eliminated, nor a mystery to be feared. It becomes information. Feedback from an intelligent system that has adapted under specific conditions. When those conditions change, the system can reorganize itself.

Yoga does not impose that change but creates the space for it. In that space, healing can begin.

# WHERE TO BEGIN: KEY TAKEAWAYS

Understanding pain is the first step, but changing how we live with the body allows healing to unfold. Recovery rarely depends on a single intervention and instead emerges from restoring safety, movement, balance, and trust within the system.

The following are some key takeaways from the book that serve as guiding principles to help the body reorganize.

### Seek Medical Evaluation When Necessary

If pain follows trauma, medical evaluation is essential. Imaging and medical care are invaluable when serious pathology must be ruled out. Understanding pain does not mean ignoring warning signs.

### Understand the Role and Limits of Medication

Pain relievers, anti-inflammatory drugs, and muscle relaxants can be helpful in acute phases. They reduce suffering and allow rest when the body is overwhelmed.

However, medication does not restore coordination, mobility, or nervous system regulation. Long-term reliance without addressing movement, posture, and lifestyle often prolongs the problem rather than resolving it. Use medication as support when needed, not as the sole solution.

### Recognize When Rest Helps and When It Harms

Short periods of rest after acute injury allow inflammation to settle. But prolonged inactivity weakens muscles, stiffens joints, and increases pain sensitivity. When rest extends beyond necessity, the body adapts to stillness. Gentle movement must be reintroduced to restore function.

### Understand Surgery as a Specific Solution, Not a Universal One

Surgical intervention can be life-changing when there is clear structural compromise. However, many spinal changes seen on imaging are part of normal aging and may not require surgery. Decisions should be made with careful consultation and full understanding of risks, benefits, and alternatives. Structure matters but function matters equally.

### Restore a Sense of Safety in the Body

Before trying to correct posture or increase flexibility, allow the nervous system to settle. Notice the breath and let it slow and soften. When breathing becomes steady, the body receives a signal that it is safe to relax. Healing begins when the system no longer feels under threat.

### Reduce Unnecessary Muscular Effort

Notice where you hold tension without awareness: in the jaw, shoulders, abdomen, or lower back. Much of this effort is habitual. Gently releasing it reduces background tension and conserves energy.

### Reintroduce Movement Gradually and Frequently

Movement nourishes discs, joints, muscles, and the nervous system. Avoiding both prolonged inactivity and sudden overexertion is important, as overdoing and underdoing are equally harmful. Move often, gently, and without urgency. Fear of movement is common after pain, but gentle, safe movement helps rebuild confidence, whereas avoidance often increases sensitivity rather than protecting the body.

### Share Effort Through the Whole Body

Allow the feet, hips, spine, and breath to participate together. When effort is distributed, no single region becomes overloaded.

### Interrupt Prolonged Sitting and Static Posture

Remaining in one position for long periods increases stiffness and pain sensitivity. Change position regularly. Even brief movement restores circulation and reduces accumulated strain.

### Let Movement Be Exploratory, Not Forceful

Avoid pushing into pain or forcing range. Move within a comfortable boundary and allow mobility to improve gradually. The nervous system responds better to safety than to force.

### Allow Time for Rest and Assimilation in Between Activity

Healing does not occur through activity alone. Periods of rest allow the nervous system to recalibrate and the body to integrate new patterns. After practice or activity, pause and allow the body to settle.

## Observe Daily Habits That Shape Pain

Posture at work, phone use, foot wear you use, kind of mattresses, breathing during stress, sleep patterns, and emotional tension all influence the spine. Healing is influenced as much by daily behavior as by formal practice. Restorative sleep supports tissue repair, nervous system regulation, and pain recovery. Improving sleep quality often improves pain tolerance and resilience.

## Stress Impacts Healing

Ongoing stress does not remain confined to the mind but it expresses itself through the body. Learning to calm the system is an essential part of physical healing.

## Practice Consistently Rather Than Intensely

Small, regular practice creates lasting adaptation. Intensity creates temporary change whereas, consistency teaches safety and resilience.

## Seek Skilled Guidance When Needed

A book can provide understanding, but healing often requires feedback and guidance. A qualified Yoga therapist, movement therapist, physiotherapist, or other skilled professional can assess movement patterns, identify compensations, guide safe progression, adapt practice to individual needs, and support confidence in movement.

There are times when self-practice is insufficient. Seeking guidance is not a failure but is an intelligent step toward recovery.

### Be Patient with the Process

Pain that developed gradually rarely disappears instantly, and healing is a progressive process. Each small improvement reflects the body's capacity to reorganize. Temporary increases in discomfort may occur as the body adapts to new patterns, but this does not necessarily indicate harm. Gradual progress, rather than constant improvement, is the natural course of healing.

### Cultivate Awareness

Awareness is the most powerful tool you possess. When you begin to notice how you move, breathe, and respond, unconscious patterns lose their hold. Change begins with noticing.

### Trust the Process

Pain is not a personal failure. It is a response shaped by experience, environment, and adaptation. Change begins not with blame, but with understanding.

Healing is not about returning to who you were. It is a gradual reorganization and discovering how the body can function with greater awareness, balance, and trust.

So, keep exploring!

# BIBLIOGRAPHY


1. Brinjikji W, Luetmer PH, Comstock B, Bresnahan BW, Chen LE, Deyo RA, et al. Systematic Literature Review of Imaging Features of Spinal Degeneration in Asymptomatic Populations. Am J Neuroradiol [Internet]. 2015 Apr 1 [cited 2026 Jan 20];36(4):811–6. Available from: https://www.ajnr.org/content/36/4/811

2. James SL, Abate D, Abate KH, Abay SM, Abbafati C, Abbasi N, et al. Global, regional, and national incidence, prevalence, and years lived with disability for 354 Diseases and Injuries for 195 countries and territories, 1990-2017: A systematic analysis for the Global Burden of Disease Study 2017. Lancet [Internet]. 2018 Nov 10 [cited 2024 Jun 5];392(10159):1789–858. Available from: http://www.thelancet.com/article/S0140673618322797/fulltext

3. Safiri S, Kolahi AA, Hoy D, Buchbinder R, Mansournia MA, Bettampadi D, et al. Global, regional, and national burden of neck pain in the general population, 1990-2017: systematic analysis of the Global Burden of Disease Study 2017. BMJ [Internet]. 2020 Mar 26 [cited 2026 Feb 4];368. Available from: https://pubmed.ncbi.nlm.nih.gov/32217608/

4. Hartvigsen J, Hancock MJ, Kongsted A, Louw Q, Ferreira ML, Genevay S, et al. What low back pain is and why we need to pay attention. Lancet [Internet]. 2018 Jun 1 [cited 2026 Feb 4];391(10137):2356–67. Available from: https://www.thelancet.com/action/showFullText?pii=S014067361830480X

5. Balagué F, Mannion AF, Pellisé F, Cedraschi C. Non-specific low back pain. Lancet [Internet]. 2012 Feb 4 [cited 2026 Feb 4];379(9814):482–91. Available from: https://www.thelancet.com/action/showFullText?pii=S0140673611606107

6. Cohen SP. Epidemiology, diagnosis, and treatment of neck pain. Mayo Clin Proc [Internet]. 2015 Feb 1 [cited 2026 Feb 4];90(2):284–99. Available from: https://pubmed.ncbi.nlm.nih.gov/25659245/

7. Yelin E, Weinstein S, King T. The burden of musculoskeletal diseases in the United States. Semin Arthritis Rheum [Internet]. 2016 Dec 1 [cited 2026 Feb 4];46(3):259–60. Available from: https://pubmed.ncbi.nlm.nih.gov/27519477/

8. Sherman KJ, Cherkin DC, Wellman RD, Cook AJ, Hawkes RJ, Delaney K, et al. A randomized trial comparing yoga, stretching, and a self-care book for chronic low back pain. Arch Intern Med [Internet]. 2011 Dec 12 [cited 2026 Feb 13];171(22):2019–26. Available from: https://pubmed.ncbi.nlm.nih.gov/22025101/

9. Hansraj KK. Assessment of Stresses in the Cervical Spine Caused by Posture and Position of the Head. [cited 2026 Feb 5]; Available from: http://www.

10. Wiech K. Deconstructing the sensation of pain: The influence of cognitive processes on pain perception. Science [Internet]. 2016 Nov 4 [cited 2026 Feb 5];354(6312):584–7. Available from: https://pubmed.ncbi.nlm.nih.gov/27811269/

11. Raja SN, Carr DB, Cohen M, Finnerup NB, Flor H, Gibson S, et al. The revised International Association for the Study of Pain definition of pain: concepts, challenges, and compromises. Pain [Internet]. 2020 Sep 1 [cited 2026 Feb 5];161(9):1976–82. Available from: https://pubmed.ncbi.nlm.nih.gov/32694387/

12. Niedenthal PM. Embodying emotion. Science [Internet]. 2007 May 18 [cited 2026 Feb 5];316(5827):1002–5. Available from: https://pubmed.ncbi.nlm.nih.gov/17510358/

13. Caggiari G, Talesa GR, Toro G, Jannelli E, Monteleone G, Puddu L. What type of mattress should be chosen to avoid back pain and improve sleep quality? Review of the literature. J Orthop Traumatol [Internet]. 2021 Dec 1 [cited 2026 Feb 5];22(1). Available from: https://pubmed.ncbi.nlm.nih.gov/34878594/

14. Kovacs FM, Abraira V, Peña A, Martín-Rodríguez JG, Sánchez-Vera M, Ferrer E, et al. Effect of firmness of mattress on chronic non-specific low-back pain: Randomised, double-blind, controlled, multicentre trial. Lancet [Internet]. 2003 Nov 15 [cited 2026 Feb 5]; 362(9396):1599–604. Available from: https://www.thelancet.com/action/showFullText?pii=S0140673603147927

15. Myrtos CD. Low Back Disorders. Evidence-Based Prevention and Rehabilitation. J Can Chiropr Assoc [Internet]. 2012 [cited 2026 Feb 5];56(1):76. Available from: https://pmc.ncbi.nlm.nih.gov/articles/PMC3280122/

16. Proske U, Gandevia SC. The proprioceptive senses: their roles in signaling body shape, body position and movement, and muscle force. Physiol Rev [Internet]. 2012 Oct 1 [cited 2026 Feb 5];92(4):1651–97. Available from: https://pubmed.ncbi.nlm.nih.gov/23073629/

17. Lieberman DE, Venkadesan M, Werbel WA, Daoud AI, Dandrea S, Davis IS, et al. Foot strike patterns and collision forces in habitually barefoot versus shod runners. Nature [Internet]. 2010 Jan 28 [cited 2026 Feb 5];463(7280):531–5. Available from: https://pubmed.ncbi.nlm.nih.gov/20111000/

18. Ridge ST, Olsen MT, Bruening DA, Jurgensmeier K, Griffin D, Davis IS, et al. Walking in Minimalist Shoes Is Effective for Strengthening Foot Muscles. Med Sci Sports Exerc [Internet]. 2019 Jan 1 [cited 2026 Feb 5];51(1):104–13. Available from: https://pubmed.ncbi.nlm.nih.gov/30113521/

19. Xie Y, Szeto G, Dai J. Prevalence and risk factors associated with musculoskeletal complaints among users of mobile handheld devices: A systematic review. Appl Ergon [Internet]. 2017 Mar 1 [cited 2026

Feb 5];59(Pt A):132–42. Available from: https://pubmed.ncbi.nlm.nih.gov/27890121/

20. Zetterberg C, Forsman M, Richter HO. Neck/shoulder discomfort due to visually demanding experimental near work is influenced by previous neck pain, task duration, astigmatism, internal eye discomfort and accommodation. PLoS One [Internet]. 2017 Aug 1 [cited 2026 Feb 5];12(8):e0182439. Available from: https://journals.plos.org/plosone/article?id=10.1371/journal.pone.0182439

21. Thayer JF, Lane RD. A model of neurovisceral integration in emotion regulation and dysregulation. J Affect Disord [Internet]. 2000 Dec 2 [cited 2026 Feb 5];61(3):201–16. Available from: https://pubmed.ncbi.nlm.nih.gov/11163422/

22. Adams MA, Dolan P. Spine biomechanics. J Biomech. 2005;38(10):1972–83.

23. Turner CH. Three rules for bone adaptation to mechanical stimuli. Bone [Internet]. 1998 Nov 1 [cited 2026 Jan 20];23(5):399–407. Available from: https://www.sciencedirect.com/science/article/abs/pii/S8756328298001185

24. Jensen MC, Brant-Zawadzki MN, Obuchowski N, Modic MT, Malkasian D, Ross JS. Magnetic Resonance Imaging of the Lumbar Spine in People without Back Pain. N Engl J Med [Internet]. 1994 Jul 14 [cited 2026 Jan 20];331(2):69–73. Available from: https://www.nejm.org/doi/pdf/10.1056/NEJM199407143310201

25. Bogduk N. Topical review On the definitions and physiology of back pain, referred pain, and radicular pain.

26. Deyo RA, Mirza SK, Turner JA, Martin BI. Overtreating Chronic Back Pain: Time to Back Off? J Am Board Fam Med [Internet]. 2009 Jan [cited 2026 Jan 20];22(1):62. Available from: https://pmc.ncbi.nlm.nih.gov/articles/PMC2729142/

27. Chou R, Qaseem A, Snow V, Casey D, Cross Jr JT, Shekelle P, et al. Diagnosis and Treatment of Low Back Pain: A Joint Clinical Practice Guideline from the American College of Physicians and the American Pain Society. https://doi.org/107326/0003-4819-147-7-200710020-00006 [Internet]. 2007 Oct 2 [cited 2026 Jan 23];147(7):478–91. Available from: /doi/pdf/10.7326/0003-4819-147-7-200710020-00006?download=true

28. Moseley GL. Reconceptualising pain according to modern pain science. Phys Ther Rev [Internet]. 2007 Sep 1 [cited 2026 Jan 22];12(3):169–78. Available from: https://www.researchgate.net/publication/233581683_Reconceptualising_pain_according_to_modern_pain_science

29. Wilgen van, Paul C, Oosterwijck V, Ittersum van. How to explain central sensitization to patients with `unexplained' chronic musculoskeletal pain: Practice guidelines. 2011 [cited 2026 Jan 22]; Available from: https://doi.org/10.1016/j.math.2011.04.005

30. Chou R, Baisden J, Carragee EJ, Resnick DK, Shaffer WO, Loeser JD. Surgery for low back pain: a review of the evidence for an American Pain Society Clinical Practice Guideline. Spine (Phila Pa 1976) [Internet]. 2009 May 1 [cited 2026 Jan 20];34(10):1094–109. Available from: https://pubmed.ncbi.nlm.nih.gov/19363455/

31. Weinstein JN, Tosteson TD, Lurie JD, Tosteson ANA, Hanscom B, Skinner JS, et al. Surgical vs Nonoperative Treatment for Lumbar Disk Herniation: The Spine Patient Outcomes Research Trial (SPORT): A Randomized Trial. JAMA [Internet]. 2006 Nov 22 [cited 2026 Jan 20];296(20):2441–50. Available from: https://jamanetwork.com/journals/jama/fullarticle/204281

32. Horak FB. Postural orientation and equilibrium: what do we need to know about neural control of balance to prevent falls? Age Ageing [Internet]. 2006 Sep 1 [cited 2026 Feb 5];35 Suppl 2(SUPPL.2). Available from: https://pubmed.ncbi.nlm.nih.gov/16926210/

33. Kleim JA, Jones TA. Principles of experience-dependent neural plasticity: implications for rehabilitation after brain damage. J Speech Lang Hear Res [Internet]. 2008 Feb 1 [cited 2026 Feb 5];51(1). Available from: https://pubmed.ncbi.nlm.nih.gov/18230848/

34. Hilibrand AS, Robbins M. Adjacent segment degeneration and adjacent segment disease: the consequences of spinal fusion? Spine J [Internet]. 2004 Nov 1 [cited 2026 Jan 20];4(6):S190–4. Available from: https://www.sciencedirect.com/science/article/abs/pii/S152994300400573X

35. Ghiselli G, Wang JC, Bhatia NN, Hsu WK, Dawson EG. This is an enhanced PDF from. J Bone Jt Surg Am J Bone Jt Surg [Internet]. 2004 [cited 2026 Jan 20];86:1497–503. Available from: www.jbjs.org

36. Bolland MJ, Grey A, Avenell A, Gamble GD, Reid IR. Calcium supplements with or without vitamin D and risk of cardiovascular events: reanalysis of the Women's Health Initiative limited access dataset and meta-analysis. BMJ [Internet]. 2011 Apr 19 [cited 2026 Jan 20];342(7804). Available from: https://www.bmj.com/content/342/bmj.d2040

37. Reid IR, Bolland MJ, Sambrook PN, Grey A. Calcium supplementation: Balancing the cardiovascular risks. Maturitas [Internet]. 2011 Aug [cited 2026 Jan 20];69(4):289–95. Available from: https://pubmed.ncbi.nlm.nih.gov/21621353/

38. Stock JT. Wolff's law (bone functional adaptation). Int Encycl Biol Anthropol [Internet]. 2018 Oct 4 [cited 2026 Jan 20];1–2. Available from: https://www.researchgate.net/publication/328111160_Wolff's_law_bone_functional_adaptation

39. Grossman DC, Curry SJ, Owens DK, Barry MJ, Caughey AB, Davidson KW, et al. Vitamin D, Calcium, or Combined Supplementation for the Primary Prevention of Fractures in Community-Dwelling Adults: US Preventive Services Task Force Recommendation Statement. JAMA [Internet]. 2018 Apr 17 [cited 2026 Feb 5];319(15):1592–9. Available from: https://jamanetwork.com/journals/jama/fullarticle/2678622

40. Yao P, Bennett D, Mafham M, Lin X, Chen Z, Armitage J, et al. Vitamin D and Calcium for the Prevention of Fracture: A Systematic Review and Meta-analysis. JAMA Netw Open [Internet]. 2019 Dec 2 [cited 2026 Feb 5];2(12):e1917789–e1917789. Available from: https://jamanetwork.com/journals/jamanetworkopen/fullarticle/2757873

41. Baigent C, Bhala N, Emberson J, Merhi A, Abramson S, Arber N, et al. Vascular and upper gastrointestinal effects of non-steroidal anti-inflammatory drugs: Meta-analyses of individual participant data from randomised trials. Lancet [Internet]. 2013 [cited 2026 Jan 23];382(9894):769–79. Available from: https://pubmed.ncbi.nlm.nih.gov/23726390/

42. Lanas A, Chan FKL. Peptic ulcer disease. Lancet [Internet]. 2017 Aug 5 [cited 2026 Jan 23];390(10094):613–24. Available from: https://pubmed.ncbi.nlm.nih.gov/28242110/

43. Van Tulder MW, Touray T, Furlan AD, Solway S, Bouter LM. Muscle relaxants for nonspecific low back pain: A systematic review within the framework of the Cochrane Collaboration. Spine (Phila Pa 1976) [Internet]. 2003 Sep 1 [cited 2026 Jan 25];28(17):1978–92. Available from: https://www.researchgate.net/publication/10568763_Muscle_Relaxants_for_Nonspecific_Low_Back_Pain_A_Systematic_Review_Within_the_Framework_of_the_Cochrane_Collaboration

44. Tulder van, Kim A, Mechelen van, and B. Occupational health guidelines for the management of low back pain: an international comparison Original Citation.

45. McKenzie R MS. The Lumbar Spine: Mechanical Diagnosis and Therapy. Spinal Publications; 2003.

46. Callaghan JP, McGill SM. Low back joint loading and kinematics during standing and unsupported sitting. Ergonomics. 2001 Feb 1;44(3):280–94.

47. American Spine Society N. Evidence-Based Clinical Guidelines for Multidisciplinary Spine Care. 2020 [cited 2026 Jan 23]; Available from: www.spine.org

48. Foster NE, Anema JR, Cherkin D, Chou R, Cohen SP, Gross DP, et al. Prevention and treatment of low back pain: evidence, challenges, and promising directions. Lancet [Internet]. 2018 Jun 9 [cited 2026 Jan 23];391(10137):2368–83. Available from: https://www.sciencedirect.com/science/article/abs/pii/S0140673618304896

49. Sherman KJ, Cherkin DC, Erro J, Miglioretti DL, Deyo RA. Comparing yoga, exercise, and a self-care book for chronic low back pain: a randomized, controlled trial. Ann Intern Med [Internet]. 2005 [cited 2026 Feb 21];143(12):849–56. Available from: https://pubmed.ncbi.nlm.nih.gov/16365466/

50. B.K.S. Iyengar. Light on the Yoga Sūtras of Patañjali. HarperCollinsPublishers; 1993.

51. Melzack R. From the gate to the neuromatrix. Pain [Internet]. 1999 [cited 2026 Feb 21];Suppl 6(SUPPL.1). Available from: https://pubmed.ncbi.nlm.nih.gov/10491980/

52. Jerath R, Edry JW, Barnes VA, Jerath V. Physiology of long pranayamic breathing: neural respiratory elements may provide a mechanism that explains how slow deep breathing shifts the autonomic nervous system. Med Hypotheses [Internet]. 2006 [cited 2026 Feb 21];67(3):566–71. Available from: https://pubmed.ncbi.nlm.nih.gov/16624497/

53. Swami Muktibodhananda. Hatha Yoga Pradipika. Yoga Publications Trust; 1998.

54. Moseley GL. Evidence for a direct relationship between cognitive and physical change during an education intervention in people with chronic low back pain. Eur J Pain [Internet]. 2004 [cited 2026 Feb 21];8(1):39–45. Available from: https://pubmed.ncbi.nlm.nih.gov/14690673/

55. Hodges PW, Tucker K. Moving differently in pain: a new theory to explain the adaptation to pain. Pain [Internet]. 2011 Mar [cited 2026 Feb 21];152(3 Suppl). Available from: https://pubmed.ncbi.nlm.nih.gov/21087823/

56. Flor H. Cortical reorganisation and chronic pain: implications for rehabilitation. J Rehabil Med [Internet]. 2003 [cited 2026 Feb 21];(41 Suppl):66–72. Available from: https://pubmed.ncbi.nlm.nih.gov/12817660/

57. Panjabi MM. The stabilizing system of the spine. Part I. Function, dysfunction, adaptation, and enhancement. J Spinal Disord [Internet]. 1992 [cited 2026 Feb 21];5(4):383–9. Available from: https://pubmed.ncbi.nlm.nih.gov/1490034/

58. Gatchel RJ, Peng YB, Peters ML, Fuchs PN, Turk DC. The biopsychosocial approach to chronic pain: scientific advances and future directions. Psychol Bull [Internet]. 2007 Jul [cited 2026 Feb 21];133(4):581–624. Available from: https://pubmed.ncbi.nlm.nih.gov/17592957/

59. McEwen BS. Physiology and neurobiology of stress and adaptation: central role of the brain. Physiol Rev [Internet]. 2007 Jul [cited 2026 Feb 21];87(3):873–904. Available from: https://pubmed.ncbi.nlm.nih.gov/17615391/

60. Streeter CC, Gerbarg PL, Saper RB, Ciraulo DA, Brown RP. Effects of yoga on the autonomic nervous system, gamma-aminobutyric-acid, and allostasis in epilepsy, depression, and post-traumatic stress disorder. Med Hypotheses [Internet]. 2012 May [cited 2026 Feb 21];78(5):571–9. Available from: https://pubmed.ncbi.nlm.nih.gov/22365651/

61. Langevin HM, Sherman KJ. Pathophysiological model for chronic low back pain integrating connective tissue and nervous system mechanisms. Med Hypotheses [Internet]. 2007 [cited 2026 Feb 21];68(1):74–80. Available from: https://pubmed.ncbi.nlm.nih.gov/16919887/

# ABOUT THE AUTHOR

Vinay Siddaiah is a Yoga practitioner, therapist, and teacher, and the founder of Yogavijnana, a center dedicated to the sincere study and practice of Yoga. His work focuses on understanding the deeper causes of physical pain through the combined perspectives of Yoga and modern science. What began as a practical solution for his back pain, soon evolved into a path of deep study, inquiry, and transformation.

Before dedicating himself fully to Yoga, Vinay served for over twelve years as a Principal Engineer in leading multinational companies. Alongside his corporate career, he spent more than a decade teaching Yoga and eventually chose to make it his life's mission.

Since 2010, Vinay has taught thousands of students, carefully observing how posture, movement, breath, emotions, and lifestyle influence the experience of back and neck pain. His approach views the body not as a machine that needs fixing, but as an intelligent system that continuously adapts and communicates.

Vinay holds a Master's degree in Yoga Therapy from SVYASA University, Bengaluru, and an M.Tech in Heritage Science and Technology from the Indian Institute of Technology (IIT) Hyderabad. He is an E-RYT 500 certified Yoga teacher with Yoga Alliance, USA.

He is also a Certified Yoga Master, Yoga Therapist and serves as a Lead examiner at Yoga Certification Board, AYUSH Ministry. He is recognized Yoga Chikitsa Acharya from Indian Yoga Association.

Through his teaching and writing, Vinay seeks to help individuals understand pain more deeply and cultivate a more intelligent relationship with their bodies.

www.ingramcontent.com/pod-product-compliance
Ingram Content Group UK Ltd.
Pitfield, Milton Keynes, MK11 3LW, UK
UKHW040232290926
15471UKWH00002B/150

9 798903 623808